Antibiotics

and the

Microbiome

How to Unlock the Healing Power
of Your Gut Microbiota to Boost
Recovery of Gut Health

PATRICK A. WALSH PhD

Disclaimer

This book is intended to supplement, not replace, the advice of a physician, pharmacist, or other trained health professionals. Always consult a trained health professional if you are unsure about your health status or the potential impact of dietary changes on your prescribed medication. The author and publisher specifically disclaim any liability, loss, or risk, personal or otherwise, that is incurred as a consequence, directly or indirectly, in the use and application of any of the contents of this book.

Identifiers:
ISBN: 978-1-9192934-0-0 (Print)
ISBN: 978-1-9192934-1-7 (eBook)

"It is health that is real wealth and not pieces of gold and silver."

— **Mahatma Gandhi**

Contents

Introduction

In recent years, the human microbiome has emerged as one of the most captivating and consequential areas of biomedical science. From bestselling books to peer-reviewed journals, the literature on the subject is now both vast and impressive. Yet, as important as these works are, they can be overwhelming for non-specialists or those looking for practical guidance rather than academic discourse. The complexity of the microbiome, while intellectually thrilling, can be a barrier to its meaningful application in daily life—especially in healthcare, education, and patient self-care. Thus, while awareness of the microbiome is growing, the challenge remains: how can individuals effectively utilize this knowledge to their benefit?

This book aims to fill that gap by offering a modest yet significant contribution to the existing body of work. Its purpose is not to compete with comprehensive academic tomes or to replace meticulous data-driven reviews; instead, it seeks to provide a condensed, accessible overview. By synthesizing key findings and actionable insights, this book is designed for a broader audience, including clinicians, educators, and individuals who wish to reclaim or maintain their health. I have distilled the essential science and presented it in a manner that is both relevant and applicable, making it easier for readers to grasp complex concepts without prior expertise. My goal is to empower readers with knowledge that can directly impact their health and well-being.

Central to the discussion is a topic that affects millions of people worldwide: the use of antibiotics and their unintended consequences on the microbiome. While antibiotics represent one of the most significant medical breakthroughs in history, saving countless lives from once fatal infections, their use comes with inherent risks. These powerful agents do not distinguish between pathogenic bacteria and the beneficial microbes that are crucial for our health. As a result, repeated or excessive exposure to antibiotics can disrupt the delicate balance of the microbiome, leading to consequences that may be transient but often result in long-lasting effects. Understanding this duality is crucial for anyone involved in healthcare or seeking to maintain their own health.

Recognizing the fragile ecology of the microbiome opens the door to new inquiries: How can we better protect the microbiome during necessary antibiotic treatments? What are the most effective methods to restore microbial diversity and resilience afterward? Moreover, what role does nutrition play in this recovery process? These questions are vital as they guide us toward empowering both patients and healthcare providers to make informed decisions based on the latest scientific research. By addressing these inquiries, we can foster a more holistic approach to health that considers the intricate relationships between antibiotics, the microbiome, and dietary choices.

This book places strong emphasis on the vital importance of supporting a healthy microbiome—not only before and during antibiotic use, but also in helping it recover afterward. It draws on current research and clinical insights to outline a multi-faceted approach to microbiome recovery—one that prioritizes diet, lifestyle, and targeted interventions over simplistic solutions. Among the most promising avenues explored is culinary medicine, an interdisciplinary field that merges the art of food preparation with the science of nutrition and preventive care. By integrating culinary medicine strategies into routine healthcare practices, providers can guide patients toward food choices that nourish not only the body but also the microbiota residing within it. This holistic approach underscores the importance of food as a fundamental component of health and recovery.

Importantly, this book serves as a valuable resource guide. Throughout its chapters, readers will find references to trusted sources in culinary medicine, educational platforms, and patient-centered tools that bridge the gap between scientific research and everyday nutrition. I highlight exemplary programs and institutions that are pioneering food-as-medicine training for healthcare professionals, as well as community-level interventions that make microbiome-supportive nutrition accessible and culturally appropriate. By providing these resources, I aim to equip readers with practical tools that can be utilized in their own lives or practices, enhancing their understanding of the microbiome's role in health.

Though simplified, the information presented in this book is firmly grounded in scientific evidence. Every effort has been made to ensure accuracy and relevance, drawing upon peer-reviewed studies, clinical guidelines, and expert opinions. Where scientific consensus exists, I emphasize it, providing readers with a clear understanding of established knowledge. Conversely, where uncertainties remain—an inherent aspect of microbiome science—I strive to present the evolving nature of the evidence with integrity and humility. This commitment to accuracy is essential, as it builds trust and empowers readers to engage with the content critically.

I recognize that readers come from diverse backgrounds and have varying interests. Healthcare providers may seek practical strategies to implement in clinical settings, while educators may look for ways to incorporate microbiome literacy into their curricula. Patients and caregivers may simply be seeking ways to improve their well-being and gain a better understanding of their health. This book aims to resonate with all these audiences, speaking to them without assuming prior expertise or requiring advanced scientific training. By doing so, I strive to create an inclusive resource that caters to the diverse needs of a broad range of readers.

Ultimately, the central message of this book is one of hope and empowerment. The microbiome is a dynamic entity that is remarkably responsive to change and influenced by our lifestyle choices. While modern life presents numerous challenges to its integrity—such as poor diet, chronic stress, environmental toxins, and medications—it is entirely possible to heal, rebuild, and support a thriving microbial community. The key lies not in seeking miracle cures but in embracing sustained, evidence-informed practices that prioritize real food, mindful living, and personalized care. This empowering perspective encourages readers to take control of their health through informed decision-making.

As we continue to unlock the mysteries of the microbiome, we are reminded of a truth both ancient and validated by modern science: we are not alone in our bodies. We exist as ecological beings, shaped by and dependent upon the intricate microbial world within us. Our health is deeply interconnected with the health of our microbiome. In caring for our microbiome, we are, in essence, caring for ourselves—impacting our immunity, digestion, moods, and overall resilience. This profound connection highlights the importance of nurturing our microbial partners as a key component of holistic health.

Chapter 1

The Microbiome

Historical Background

The belief that food plays a foundational role in human health is as ancient as the practice of medicine itself. Across various civilizations, food has been regarded not just as a means of sustenance but also as a primary tool for healing and disease prevention. Historical practices, such as the dietary prescriptions of Traditional Chinese Medicine and Ayurveda, along with Hippocrates' enduring maxim, "Let food be thy medicine," highlight the longstanding interplay between diet and well-being. For centuries, early medical traditions emphasized concepts like balance, digestion, and the energetic properties of food, providing a framework for health practices. However, our early ancestors developed these practices without any understanding of the microscopic world residing within them, a world that would later prove crucial to their health.

The scientific advances of the 19th and 20th centuries finally brought the invisible agents of health and disease—microorganisms—into view. Initially, these tiny entities were understood primarily as pathogens responsible for illness and infection. Over time, groundbreaking research, particularly the pioneering work of Élie Metchnikoff, revolutionized this perspective. Metchnikoff introduced the concept that beneficial bacteria, especially those found in fermented foods, could enhance health and promote longevity. Although his ideas faced skepticism initially, they laid the groundwork for our contemporary understanding of probiotics and gut ecology, fundamentally altering how we perceive the relationship between diet and health.

Today, the field of microbiome research has shed light on the integral role our microbial partners play in our overall health. The human gut is now recognized as a dynamic and diverse ecosystem that hosts trillions of microbes, which influence various aspects of our physiology, including metabolism, immune regulation, mood, and other physiological processes. Importantly, our diet serves as the most powerful lever we possess to shape this microbial ecosystem. The choices we make regarding food—not only what we consume but also how we prepare and process it—have a profound impact on the diversity and functionality of our gut microbiota. This evolving understanding has given rise to the relatively new field of culinary medicine, which merges the art of cooking with the science of nutrition. Culinary medicine emphasizes personalized, practical, and microbiome-friendly eating approaches. By revisiting ancient dietary wisdom through the lens of modern microbiology, culinary medicine creates a renewed framework for utilizing food as a therapeutic tool, acknowledging the intricate cultural and biological complexities involved in our eating habits. The historical journey from ancient food philosophies to contemporary microbiome research highlights a timeless truth: what we eat fundamentally shapes who we are, down to our microbial core.

What is the Microbiome?

The term microbiome refers to the entire habitat, including the microorganisms (bacteria, viruses, fungi, and archaea), their genomes, and the environmental conditions that exist in that habitat[1]. The organisms making up the microbiome are often collectively referred to as the microbiota or flora. The collection of genomes from the members of the microbiota constitutes what is known as the metagenome.

The genome of a single symbiotic microbial species is thought to be insufficient for its survival. However, through metabolic networks and cross-feeding, microbiota can survive as interdependent communities in their respective habitats[2].

Microbiota reside in various areas, including the skin, mouth, nasal passages, respiratory tract, urogenital tract, and most significantly, the gastrointestinal tract. The total bacterial biomass residing in and on adult humans is estimated to be approximately 200 grams, of which about 100 grams of bacteria comprise the gut microbiome[3]. Studies have shown that the ratio of bacteria to human cells is approximately 4×10^{13} bacterial cells to 3×10^{13} human cells, resulting in a near 1:1 ratio[4]. This intricate community plays essential roles in our physiology and health and is crucial for human life.

The latest metagenomic analysis of 11,850 human gut microbiomes from diverse countries and ethnic backgrounds has identified 1,952 distinct uncultured candidate bacterial species[1, 5]. Of the total number of identified bacterial species, each individual typically harbors around 150–400 species[4, 6-8]. This considerable inter-individual variability in microbiome composition can be attributed to a variety of factors, including host genetics, mode of delivery (vaginal vs. cesarean delivery), diet, geographic location, lifestyle choices, age, and the use of antibiotics or other medications[9-12].

The influence of the human host genome on gut microbiota appears to be minimal. Evidence from both population studies across various ethnic groups and twin studies involving over 1,000 pairs suggests that only 2-9% of the microbial taxa found in stool samples of adults appear to be heritable[11, 13].

Of the multitude of environmental factors that have been investigated, diet has been recognized as one of the most influential ecological determinants of microbial populations. For example, individuals who consume a high-fiber, plant-based diet tend to harbor more diverse and beneficial microbial communities compared to those who follow a Western diet, high in fat and sugar, underscoring the crucial role of diet in shaping our microbial landscape.

Microbiome and Evolving Research Technologies

The study of microorganisms dates back to the 17th century when Antonie van Leeuwenhoek, using a handmade microscope, first observed "animalcules" present in water and human saliva. This marked an early glimpse into the complex world of microbes. However, it would take centuries for a more comprehensive understanding of how these microbes interact with human health to emerge. The modern field of microbiome research began to flourish in the early 2000s, driven by revolutionary advances in DNA sequencing technologies, including 16S ribosomal RNA gene sequencing and metagenomics. These innovations enabled scientists to identify and characterize microbes directly from environmental or human samples, thereby eliminating the reliance on traditional culturing techniques[14].

In 2007, the Human Microbiome Project (HMP)[15] was launched, funded by the U.S. National Institutes of Health, to map the microbial ecosystems of healthy individuals. This landmark project revealed that microbial diversity varies not only between individuals but also across different sites within the same body. Moreover, it established a foundational understanding that disruptions in microbial balance, referred to as dysbiosis, are associated with a wide range of health conditions. These include inflammatory bowel disease, obesity, allergies, diabetes, and mental health disorders such as depression and anxiety[16]. The insights gained from the HMP have been pivotal in advancing microbiome research.

Epilogue

Today, microbiome science is one of the fastest-growing fields in biomedical research. Scientists are actively exploring personalized microbiome therapies, probiotics, and dietary interventions to modulate microbial communities and improve health outcomes. As our knowledge deepens, the microbiome is reshaping our understanding of the human body, not merely as a standalone organism, but as a complex ecosystem in constant dialogue with its microbial inhabitants. This shift in perspective underlines the importance of the microbiome in maintaining health and preventing disease.

Chapter 2

The Microbial World Within

Overview of the Gastrointestinal Tract

The human gastrointestinal tract extends from the esophagus to the anus, with each section differing in length and microbial composition. The esophagus, which is roughly 25 cm long, primarily harbors transient microbes from the oral cavity. The stomach, approximately 20–30 cm in length and holding 1–1.5 liters, maintains a highly acidic environment, which limits the density of microorganisms. Nevertheless, acid-tolerant genera are present. The small intestine spans approximately 6 meters and is divided into the duodenum (25–30 cm), jejunum (2.5 m), and ileum (3.5 m). The duodenum has relatively few bacteria due to the presence of bile and pancreatic secretions. The jejunum supports modest populations, while the ileum, being closer to the colon, houses denser communities. The large intestine (colon) measures about 1.5 meters and is the most densely populated microbial niche in the body, reaching up to 10^{12} cells per gram of content. Here, strict anaerobic bacterial communities predominate, forming the core of the gut microbiome. Finally, the rectum and anus, which are approximately 12–15 cm in combined length, serve as the terminal reservoir and exit point. Their microbial communities resemble those of the distal colon, enriched in anaerobes adapted to low-oxygen environments.

Types of Microbes in the Gut Microbiome

The human gastrointestinal tract is home to a dense and diverse microbial ecosystem, commonly referred to as the gut microbiome. This ecosystem is foundational not only for digestion but also for immune modulation, nutrient synthesis, and overall health. While bacteria dominate in terms of abundance and research focus, other microbial groups—including viruses, fungi, and archaea—also play crucial roles in maintaining the functional complexity and resilience of the gut microbiome. Understanding the various types of microbes within this complex environment is essential for appreciating their contributions to health.

Bacteria constitute the most extensively studied and abundant component of the gut microbiota. Of the 55 phyla that comprise the domain Bacteria, only seven to nine are found in the human gut, with the majority (approximately 90%) belonging to the *Bacteroidetes* and

Firmicutes phyla, respectively[17]. Other phyla found in the gut include *Actinobacteria, Fusobacteria, Proteobacteria*, and *Verrucomicrobia*. However, it is essential to recognize that not all gut bacteria are beneficial. Opportunistic pathogens, such as *Clostridium difficile,* can proliferate when microbial balance is disrupted, commonly following antibiotic use, leading to severe gastrointestinal infections. This highlights the importance of maintaining microbial equilibrium for overall health. Maintaining a balanced gut microbiome is crucial for preventing diseases and promoting a healthy digestive environment.

The gut also houses a vast population of **viruses**, collectively known as the **virome**. Most of these are bacteriophages—viruses that specifically infect and replicate within bacteria. Bacteriophages play a significant role in shaping microbial communities by lysing specific bacterial hosts, thereby influencing bacterial diversity and abundance. Emerging research suggests that the virome may also modulate host immune responses and metabolic pathways, although studies in this area are still in their infancy[18]. The dynamic nature of the gut virome and its impact on overall gut health are areas of ongoing research.

Though present in smaller populations, **fungi**—referred to as the **mycobiome**—also inhabit the gut. Common fungal genera include *Candida, Saccharomyces*, and *Malassezia*. Under normal circumstances, these fungi coexist harmoniously with other microbes. However, in situations where fungal populations overgrow—often as a result of antibiotic use or immune suppression—they can contribute to dysbiosis, inflammation, and gastrointestinal discomfort[19]. For instance, *Candida albicans* is notable for its ability to transition from a benign yeast form to an invasive filamentous form, which can trigger immune responses and exacerbate intestinal inflammation in vulnerable individuals.

Archaea represent a distinct domain of life, separate from bacteria and eukaryotes. In the human gut, their presence is less abundant yet functionally significant. The most prominent archaeal species is *Methanobrevibacter smithii,* which aids digestion by consuming hydrogen produced during fermentation and converting it into methane[20]. This metabolic process helps maintain fermentation efficiency and may influence gut transit time and bloating. Although archaea typically do not elicit immune responses, changes in their abundance have been linked to metabolic conditions, including obesity and irritable bowel syndrome, suggesting that their broader roles in host health may be more critical than previously understood.

Together, these various microbes form a complex, interdependent network, akin to a bustling city. They interact, compete, and cooperate in ways that significantly influence digestion, immunity, metabolism, and neurological health. Understanding these interactions is crucial for comprehending how the microbiome influences our overall well-being and how we can manipulate it to achieve better health outcomes.

How Microbes Colonize the Human Body

The ecological dynamics of the human gut microbiome undergo rapid changes during early childhood, particularly between the ages of 0 and 3. This period is characterized by significant changes as the gut microbiome begins to establish itself, influenced by a multitude of factors, including the mode of delivery (vaginal vs. cesarean), gestational age at birth, exposure to antibiotics, infant feeding practices (breastfeeding versus formula feeding), the timing and type of solid food introduction, contact with animals, environmental exposures, number of siblings, and psychological stress[9, 21-26]. During these formative years, the diversity and composition of gut bacteria are shaped, laying the foundation for an individual's health and immune system. At age three, a child's gut microbiome typically resembles that of an adult.

Breastfeeding plays a pivotal role in shaping the infant's gut microbiome during the early stages of life. Human milk serves not only as a source of essential nutrients but also as a complex bioactive fluid that significantly contributes to microbial colonization and the development of the immune system[27]. One of the key components of breast milk is human milk oligosaccharides (HMOs), a diverse group of complex carbohydrates that are indigestible by infants but serve as selective substrates for beneficial gut bacteria, particularly *Bifidobacterium longum subsp. Infantis (B. Infantis)*[28, 29]. HMOs promote the growth of *B. infantis*, which is crucial for developing a healthy gut ecosystem by outcompeting potential pathogens, modulating immune responses, and enhancing intestinal barrier function.

In addition to HMOs, breast milk contains live bacteria that further enrich the infant's microbiota. These bacteria include species from the genera *Streptococcus, Staphylococcus, Lactobacillus, and Bifidobacterium,* which are believed to be transferred from the maternal gut and skin through an entero-mammary pathway[30]. The microbial composition of breastfed infants tends to be less diverse but is enriched in beneficial taxa compared to formula-fed infants. This enriched microbiota is associated with improved resistance to infections, a lower risk of allergies, and better long-term metabolic outcomes[31]. Collectively, breastfeeding acts as a natural inoculum and nutrient source that optimally supports early microbial and immune development in infants.

Following the dynamic phase of early childhood, the gut microbiome enters a prolonged stage of relative stability, during which the established microbial community becomes more resilient and consistent. However, as individuals age, especially in their later years, the microbiome undergoes gradual changes, reflecting the ongoing evolution of the gut ecosystem.

In individuals aged 65 and above, recent studies have revealed several significant connections between gut microbiome composition and various health factors, including physical fitness, frailty, and dietary habits[32]. This growing body of research underscores the pivotal role that gut microbiome health plays in later stages of life, where maintaining a balanced microbial community can have a profound impact on overall well-being. As people age, alterations in diet, lifestyle, and physiological changes can lead to shifts in microbiome diversity, which may contribute to the development of age-related health issues. Understanding these relationships can inform strategies for promoting gut health in older adults, potentially enhancing their quality of life[33].

Studies of the gut microbiota composition in individuals aged 100 years or older (centenarians) have revealed significant differences between centenarians and other age groups. In particular, centenarians show an abundance of four main types of gut bacteria, including *Akkermansia muciniphila, Odoribacter splanchnicus, Oscillibacter sphaeroides,* and *Christensenella minuta*[34, 35]. These bacteria are linked to improved immune function, reduced inflammation, better metabolic health, and enhanced cognitive function.

An Overview of the Functions of the Gut Microbiota

The gut microbiota possess a large collective genome (the microbiome) that encodes many metabolic capabilities absent in the human genome. In the gut, these microorganisms aid in digesting dietary components (fibers, resistant starches, plant polyphenols) that the human body cannot break down on its own. They degrade host-derived glycans and mucin when needed. They modulate energy balance, fat storage, and appetite. They are responsible for producing essential nutrients, such as vitamin K and several B vitamins, which are crucial for various bodily functions. Furthermore, the gut microbiota modulates the immune system and helps prevent the colonization of the gut by pathogenic organisms[36]. Increasing evidence also suggests that the gut microbiome communicates with several other organ systems throughout the body, including the brain, endocrine system, and lungs. For example, the gut-brain axis has been identified as a pathway through which the gut can influence mood, cognition, and behavior, which is why the gut is often referred to as the "second brain"[37]. All of these functions are central to normal physiology; disruptions (dysbiosis) are increasingly implicated in metabolic, inflammatory, and other diseases.

Epilogue

In a healthy state, the upper adult human gut contains few microbes, whereas the colon supports dense communities ($>10^{12}$ per gram), forming the core microbiome. It is a diverse ecosystem of bacteria, viruses, fungi, and archaea that supports digestion, immunity, and overall health. Microbial colonization begins at birth and is influenced by early-life factors, such as delivery mode and feeding practices, with breastfeeding playing a crucial role in promoting the growth of beneficial bacteria. After early childhood, the microbiome stabilizes but continues to undergo further changes with age. In older adults, its composition is linked to physical fitness, diet, and frailty. These findings underscore the lifelong impact of the microbiome and emphasize the importance of maintaining its balance to support overall health throughout the lifespan.

Chapter 3

The Microbiome as an Endocrine Organ

Introduction

Traditionally, an endocrine organ is defined as a tissue that generates signaling molecules, commonly known as hormones, which are released into the bloodstream to regulate the functions of distant target organs. The microbiome meets these classical criteria by performing several key functions. Firstly, it produces various hormone-like substances that can influence host physiology. Secondly, it modulates the synthesis of host hormones, thereby affecting hormonal balance. Lastly, the microbiome interacts with endocrine glands through a combination of neural, immune, and chemical signaling pathways. This recognition of the microbiome as an active endocrine organ transforms our understanding, shifting the perspective from viewing it as a passive assemblage of gut flora to recognizing it as a vital participant in systemic regulatory mechanisms.

The human microbiome is increasingly understood as a crucial component of the body's endocrine system. As an endocrine organ, the microbiome engages in complex bidirectional communication with the host through the synthesis, metabolism, and modulation of hormones, neurotransmitters, and various signaling molecules[38]. This dynamic interaction allows the microbiome to play a pivotal role in regulating essential physiological processes, encompassing metabolism, mood, appetite, inflammation, and even behavior[37, 39]. By understanding the microbiome's endocrine functions, we can appreciate its influence on overall health and well-being.

Short-Chain Fatty Acids (SCFAs)

Short-chain fatty acids (SCFAs) are saturated aliphatic organic acids with fewer than six carbon atoms, primarily produced through the fermentation of dietary fibers by anaerobic gut microbiota in the colon. The most abundant SCFAs are acetate (C2), propionate (C3), and butyrate (C4), which together account for over 95% of total SCFAs in the gut lumen. The SCFAs have many vital functions within the body. They are an essential energy source for host cells, particularly in the colon, providing 60–70% of the energy requirement of colon epithelial cells in humans.

They also have potent anti-inflammatory properties and help maintain gut barrier function by regulating gut permeability and the expression of tight junction proteins. Butyrate, specifically, has been shown to enhance the intestinal barrier[40].

SCFAs as Signaling Molecules

SCFAs serve as important signaling molecules that influence various endocrine pathways within the body. They achieve this by binding to G-protein-coupled receptors, specifically GPR41 and GPR43, located on enteroendocrine cells in the gut. This interaction stimulates the release of hormones such as glucagon-like peptide-1 (GLP-1) and peptide YY (PYY), both of which play crucial roles in regulating insulin secretion, appetite, and gut motility[41, 42]. Furthermore, SCFAs are capable of crossing the blood-brain barrier, enabling them to influence central nervous system signaling and thereby reinforce the microbiome's potential as an endocrine organ[43].

Thus, it can be concluded that the multifaceted influence of SCFAs underscores their importance as mediators between diet, microbial ecology, and host physiology.

Neurotransmitter Synthesis

The gut is a significant source of neurotransmitters, which are chemical messengers crucial for communication throughout the body. A diverse range of gut bacteria are known to synthesize classical neurotransmitters, contributing to the complex interplay between the microbiome and the nervous system. For instance, approximately 90% of serotonin, a crucial neurotransmitter that regulates mood and behavior, is produced in the gut, primarily by enterochromaffin cells that are stimulated by microbial metabolites. Specific species of spore-forming Clostridia have been shown to promote serotonin biosynthesis, underscoring the microbiome's impact on mental health[44, 45]. Additionally, gut bacteria such as *Lactobacillus* and *Bifidobacterium* species produce gamma-aminobutyric acid (GABA), which modulates stress and anxiety pathways[46]. Other species, including *Escherichia*, *Bacillus*, and *Saccharomyces*, can convert precursors into catecholamines such as dopamine and norepinephrine, which can influence gut motility and possibly central nervous system functions[47]. These neurotransmitters exert localized effects within the gut and can also influence systemic physiological states through pathways such as the vagus nerve or the bloodstream.

The Gut-Brain-Endocrine Axis

The microbiome is an integral part of the gut-brain-endocrine axis. From a functional perspective, the system is often described as consisting of two components: the gut-brain axis (GBA) and the hypothalamic-pituitary-adrenal axis (HPA).

The gut-brain axis is a critical and dynamic communication system that governs numerous aspects of both physical and mental health. Disruptions to this axis, caused by poor diet, stress, infections, or antibiotic use, can lead to both gastrointestinal and neuropsychiatric disorders.

The **gut-brain axis (GBA)** represents a complex, bidirectional exchange network that connects the gastrointestinal tract and the central nervous system (CNS). This intricate system encompasses a variety of pathways, including neural, hormonal, immune, and microbial channels, ensuring ongoing communication between the gut and the brain. Gaining insight into the GBA is essential for understanding its vital role in maintaining homeostasis and its effects on various physiological and psychological processes. The interaction between these systems has attracted significant attention, impacting everything from digestion to emotional regulation[48]. Research into GBA is revealing the significant ways gut health can influence mental well-being and vice versa.

At the heart of the gut-brain axis is the vagus nerve, the tenth cranial nerve that acts as a primary pathway for transmitting neural signals between the gut and the brain. Notably, around 80–90% of the fibers within the vagus nerve are afferent, carrying sensory information from the gut to the brain. This structural characteristic underscores the crucial role of the vagus nerve in regulating various bodily functions, including digestion, satiety, inflammation, and emotional responses[49]. Supporting the vagus nerve's function is the enteric nervous system (ENS), often referred to as the "second brain". The ENS consists of over 100 million neurons located in the walls of the gastrointestinal tract and functions independently of the CNS, showing sensitivity to psychological stress and influencing gut motility, secretion, and local immune responses[50].

Research has increasingly demonstrated strong links between the gut microbiome and mental health, with influences communicated through the gut-brain axis[38]. Patients suffering from depression often exhibit dysbiosis, resulting in a loss of gut microbial diversity and a decrease in beneficial bacteria, such as *Lactobacillus* and *Bifidobacterium*. In a compelling study, fecal microbiota from depressed patients were transferred to germ-free mice, resulting in depressive-like behavior in the mice, suggesting a direct causal relationship between microbiota and mood. Furthermore, individuals suffering from anxiety or chronic stress frequently show elevated markers of gut inflammation, accompanied by altered microbiota composition[51]. These findings confirm the critical role of gut health in mental well-being and highlight the potential of microbiome-targeted therapies.

Psychobiotics refer to beneficial bacteria, or probiotics, as well as prebiotics that can influence mental health through the gut-brain axis[47]. Certain strains, such as *Lactobacillus rhamnosus* and *Bifidobacterium longum*, have demonstrated promising effects in reducing symptoms of anxiety and depression in both animal models and human clinical trials. These interventions may function by restoring microbial balance, enhancing SCFA production, reducing inflammation, and modulating neurotransmitter levels. By targeting the gut microbiome, these strategies have the potential to improve mental health outcomes and provide new avenues for treatment. The growing interest in psychobiotics highlights the interconnection between gut health and mental well-being, paving the way for future research and therapeutic applications.

Recent research has been carried out, exploring the influence of gut microbiota on neurodevelopmental conditions such as autism spectrum disorder (ASD) and attention-deficit/hyperactivity disorder (ADHD). Children with ASD often exhibit gastrointestinal symptoms alongside altered microbial profiles[52]. In pilot studies, microbiota transfer therapy has shown promise in improving both gastrointestinal and behavioral symptoms in children diagnosed with ASD. Moreover, gut bacteria may play a role in cognition and brain plasticity. In experiments with mice, depletion of the microbiome impaired learning and memory, whereas reintroducing specific microbial strains reversed these cognitive deficits[53]. These findings suggest that the gut microbiome may influence cognitive development and function, highlighting its significance in neurodevelopmental disorders.

The **hypothalamic-pituitary-adrenal (HPA) axis** serves as a central stress-response system within the body. Dysbiosis can lead to an overactive HPA axis, resulting in elevated levels of cortisol and heightened stress responses[54]. In contrast, a healthy gut microbiota has been shown to buffer stress by moderating HPA axis activity, allowing for a more balanced response to stressors. Research involving germ-free mice has demonstrated that the absence of gut microbiota results in exaggerated HPA responses to stress. This effect can be normalized through microbial colonization, particularly with the administration of *Bifidobacterium infantis*[54]. This highlights the importance of maintaining a balanced gut microbiome for effective stress regulation.

The Gut–Lung Axis: How Gut Health Shapes Breathing

Scientists increasingly recognize a two-way "gut–lung axis" that links intestinal health with respiratory function. One important mechanism involves short-chain fatty acids (SCFAs), which are produced when gut bacteria ferment dietary fiber. These SCFAs travel through the bloodstream and can interact with immune cells in the lungs, thereby reducing excessive inflammation[55]. For example, animal studies have shown that a high-fiber diet increases SCFAs and helps protect against allergic airway inflammation.

When the gut microbiome is out of balance, known as dysbiosis, the immune system may overreact, leading to lung issues. Research has shown that early disruptions in gut bacteria can increase the risk of asthma. At the same time, individuals with chronic lung diseases such as COPD and cystic fibrosis often exhibit abnormal gut microbial patterns[56]. Significantly, this communication goes both ways: serious respiratory infections, such as influenza, can also disrupt gut microbial balance, which further weakens the body's defenses.

Scientific studies provide clear examples of the gut–lung axis functioning. In one study, infants who later developed asthma had lower diversity of gut bacteria early in life. Transferring those missing microbes into mice reduced airway inflammation, indicating a causal link between gut microbes and lung immunity[56]. Other research confirms that microbial signals from the gut influence the development of T cells, cytokines, and other immune messengers that are essential for lung health.

An emerging area of interest is whether acupuncture, a traditional therapy, can influence this axis. Recent studies suggest that acupuncture can modulate inflammation and rebalance immune responses[57]. A systematic review found that acupuncture treatments in both animals and humans help restore a healthier gut microbiota, with improvements observed in conditions such as irritable bowel syndrome and depression[57].

This suggests that acupuncture could indirectly support lung health by stabilizing gut flora. A clinical trial currently underway in China is exploring this idea: researchers are examining whether acupuncture improves symptoms in patients with chronic obstructive pulmonary disease (COPD) by altering gut microbiota, microbial metabolites, and immune activity[58]. The findings may help determine if traditional acupuncture benefits respiratory diseases through mechanisms aligned with the gut–lung axis.

In Traditional Chinese Medicine (TCM), Stomach-36 (ST36) is a well-known acupuncture point on the stomach meridian, often used to enhance both digestion and respiratory resilience, reflecting an ancient understanding of the gut–lung interdependence. While modern science and traditional practices speak different languages, both agree that gut health is vital for good breathing.

In conclusion, a healthy gut microbiome supports lung health by reducing inflammation and training immune cells, whereas dysbiosis increases susceptibility to asthma and infections. Acupuncture, by influencing gut microbes and immunity, could offer a new way to strengthen this connection. Although more clinical studies are needed, one thing is clear: taking care of gut health also means taking care of your breath.

Bile Acid Metabolism and Endocrine Crosstalk

Gut microbes play a crucial role in converting primary bile acids into secondary bile acids, including deoxycholic acid and lithocholic acid. These secondary bile acids serve as signaling molecules that bind to specific receptors, such as the farnesoid X receptor (FXR) and the G-protein-coupled bile acid receptor (TGR5)[59]. By engaging these receptors, secondary bile acids can influence insulin sensitivity, energy expenditure, and inflammatory status within the body. This intricate crosstalk between bile acids and microbial activity highlights the microbiome's significant role in regulating host metabolism through bile acid signaling, a fundamental endocrine function[60]. Understanding these interactions offers valuable insights into how the microbiome influences metabolic health and disease.

Modulation of Hormonal Function and Metabolism

The **estrobolome**[61], a specialized subset of the microbiota, contains genes that metabolize estrogens, thereby impacting systemic estrogen levels through processes such as deconjugation and enterohepatic recycling. Disruption of the estrobolome has been linked to various estrogen-driven conditions, including endometriosis, polycystic ovarian syndrome (PCOS), and breast cancer. In addition to influencing sex hormones, gut microbes also play a vital role in the production and clearance of metabolic hormones. These include insulin, which regulates blood sugar levels; leptin, involved in appetite regulation; ghrelin, known as the hunger hormone; and thyroid hormones, which are crucial for metabolism. For instance, dysbiosis, an imbalance in gut microbiota, has been linked to insulin resistance, underscoring the microbiome's endocrine relevance in metabolic disorders, such as type 2 diabetes[62]. The importance of gut microbiota in normalizing insulin function is further substantiated by studies showing that the transfer of intestinal microbiota from lean donors increases insulin sensitivity in individuals with metabolic syndrome[63]. This connection highlights the significance of maintaining a healthy microbiome for achieving hormonal balance and optimal metabolic health.

Epilogue

The human microbiome fulfills every functional criterion of an endocrine organ. It produces and modulates hormones and signaling molecules, affects distant organ systems, and integrates with classical endocrine pathways. Its influence spans from metabolism and immunity to neurological and psychological health. Recognizing the microbiome as an endocrine organ not only enhances our understanding of systemic physiology but also opens new avenues for diagnostics, preventive medicine, and therapeutic strategies in a wide range of chronic diseases.

Chapter 4

The Microbiome and the Immune System

Introduction

The human immune system is immature at birth and undergoes significant postnatal development, heavily influenced by exposure to microbes. Germ-free (GF) mouse models have been pivotal in understanding this relationship. GF mice display underdeveloped lymphoid tissues, including smaller Peyer's patches and mesenteric lymph nodes, reduced populations of regulatory T cells (Tregs), and impaired immunoglobulin A (IgA) secretion. Colonization of GF mice with normal microbiota reverses many of these deficiencies, underscoring the essential role of microbiota in immune maturation[64].

The development of the immune system during the early stages of life is crucial as infants transition from the protected environment of the womb to a world where their immune system must operate, adapt, and demonstrate resilience. In the first days and weeks after birth, infants are particularly vulnerable to infections because their immune systems are still developing. Over time, the infant's immune system needs to learn to defend against harmful pathogens while also identifying and accepting non-threatening substances[65]. This adaptive process is tightly orchestrated and occurs in tandem with colonization by maternal and environmental microbes.

Approximately 70–80% of immune cells are located in the gut, particularly within the intestinal epithelium, the innermost layer of cells[66]. This layer, characterized by extensive folding and the considerable length of the intestines, serves as the body's most significant and crucial interface with the outside environment. The epithelial barrier not only protects against pathogens but also serves as a hub for immunological activities, housing a dense concentration of immune cells and tissues. Central to this interface is the human gut microbiome, a complex ecosystem comprising trillions of bacteria, viruses, fungi, and archaea, all of which play a vital role in shaping and regulating the immune system. Far from being a passive collection of microbes, the gut microbiome engages in dynamic, bidirectional communication with both innate and adaptive branches of the immune system. This interaction is particularly evident in the gut-associated lymphoid tissue (GALT), where immune cells regularly sample microbial antigens to promote immune education, tolerance to beneficial microbes, and defense against harmful pathogens. Therefore, the gut epithelium, immune system, and microbiome form a closely linked triad that is essential for sustaining health and homeostasis.

GALT: The Frontline of Immune-Microbial Interaction

The gut-associated lymphoid tissue (GALT) comprises specialized immune structures that play a crucial role in the body's defense mechanisms. These structures include Peyer's patches, isolated lymphoid follicles, and mesenteric lymph nodes. Each of these components functions as a sentinel site, capable of detecting and responding to microbial components and food antigens. By recognizing these elements, GALT ensures that the immune system can effectively differentiate between harmful pathogens and beneficial substances. This proactive response is essential for maintaining overall gut health and the body's immune equilibrium.

Within the GALT, microfold (M) cells are responsible for transporting microbial antigens from the intestinal lumen to antigen-presenting cells (APCs), which primarily include dendritic cells (DCs). Once these DCs receive the antigens, they activate naive T cells and B cells, which then differentiate into specific immune cells. A significant outcome of this process is the production of immunoglobulin A (IgA), which binds to gut microbes and plays a protective role by preventing their translocation across the epithelial barrier. This mechanism is particularly crucial because secretory IgA helps maintain mucosal homeostasis while avoiding inflammatory responses that could lead to tissue damage. Thus, the actions of M cells and DCs are essential for the gut's immune function and overall health.

Commensal microbes are integral to the maturation of GALT and play a key role in modulating epithelial integrity. For instance, the bacterium *Bacteroides fragilis* produces polysaccharide A (PSA), which interacts with Toll-like receptor 2 (TLR2) on dendritic cells, inducing regulatory T cell responses and suppressing inflammation. The presence of such beneficial microbes supports the gut's structural and functional integrity, contributing to a balanced immune response. Overall, the relationship between commensal bacteria and GALT highlights the complexity of gut microbiota interactions and their impact on immune health[67].

Regulatory T Cells (Tregs) and Immune Tolerance

Regulatory T cells (Tregs) play a crucial role in maintaining immune homeostasis by suppressing excessive immune responses and promoting tolerance to self and non-harmful antigens. Their development and function depend on the expression of FOXP3, a transcription factor encoded by the FOXP3 gene, often referred to as the "master regulator" of T regulatory cells (Tregs).

The gut microbiota significantly influences Treg differentiation, particularly in the colon. This is primarily mediated through microbial metabolites, especially short-chain fatty acids (SCFAs) such as butyrate and propionate. These SCFAs are fermentation products of dietary fiber by gut bacteria, promoting the differentiation of naïve T cells into colonic T regulatory cells (Tregs)[68]. Similarly, researchers have observed that germ-free (GF) mice have drastically reduced colonic Treg populations, a deficit that is corrected upon colonization with SCFA-producing microbes[69].

Certain bacterial strains, such as *Clostridia clusters IV and XIVa*, are particularly effective at inducing colonic Tregs. These beneficial microbes create a tolerogenic environment by stimulating epithelial cells and antigen-presenting cells to secrete anti-inflammatory mediators such as interleukin-10 (IL-10) and transforming growth factor-beta (TGF-β). These mediators are crucial for enhancing Treg-mediated suppression of effector T cells, thereby ensuring that the immune response remains balanced and under control. By promoting Treg development and function, these microbial strains contribute to maintaining gut homeostasis and preventing autoimmune conditions[70].

Thus, the relationship between the gut microbiome and Treg cells is a cornerstone of mucosal immunity.

SCFA-producing microbes, especially Clostridia clusters IV and XIVa, not only enhance *FOXP3* expression but also cultivate a cytokine environment conducive to Treg differentiation and function. These interactions are vital for suppressing inflammation, promoting tolerance to dietary and microbial antigens, and preventing autoimmune diseases. Disruption in this axis can contribute to disorders such as inflammatory bowel disease, allergies, and other autoimmune conditions.

Innate Immunity and Microbial Recognition

The Innate immune system provides the first line of defense. Innate immunity in the gut relies on various pattern recognition receptors (PRRs), such as Toll-like receptors (TLRs) and NOD-like receptors (NLRs), which are designed to detect microbial-associated molecular patterns (MAMPs)[71]. These receptors are expressed by intestinal epithelial cells, macrophages, and dendritic cells, enabling them to effectively distinguish between commensal and pathogenic microbes. This capability is crucial for initiating appropriate immune responses while preventing unnecessary inflammation from harmless microbes. By recognizing specific microbial signatures, the innate immune system can tailor its responses to maintain gut health. The intricate balance maintained by these receptors is vital for overall immune function and disease prevention. Furthermore, commensal bacteria stimulate TLR signaling, which helps promote the production of antimicrobial peptides and mucin, thereby strengthening gut barrier integrity.

When TLRs are activated by microbial ligands, such as lipopolysaccharide (LPS) from Gram-negative bacteria or flagellin from motile bacteria, they trigger signaling cascades that result in the production of pro-inflammatory cytokines and antimicrobial peptides. This process is essential for mounting an effective defense against infections. However, chronic overactivation of TLRs, which can occur due to dysbiosis, may lead to pathological inflammation, as observed in conditions like inflammatory bowel disease (IBD). This highlights the dual role of TLRs in both protecting the host and potentially contributing to disease when their regulation is disrupted.

Commensal microbes also play a significant role in regulating the function of innate lymphoid cells, specifically Group 3 Innate Lymphoid Cells (ILC3s), which are abundant in the gut. These cells produce interleukin-22 (IL-22), a cytokine crucial for maintaining epithelial barrier function and stimulating the production of antimicrobial peptides. Dysbiosis, or microbial imbalance, can impair the function of ILC3s, leading to increased susceptibility to intestinal pathogens. This illustrates the interconnectedness of the microbiome and innate immune responses, where disruptions in microbial communities can have profound effects on immune system efficacy. The proper functioning of ILC3s is thus crucial for protecting against infections and maintaining gut health[72].

Adaptive Immunity: Education by the Microbiome

The adaptive immune system, composed of B and T lymphocytes, exhibits remarkable plasticity and specificity in response to microbial antigens in the gut. These interactions are vital for shaping long-term immune memory and for maintaining mucosal homeostasis.

Peyer's patches are specialized lymphoid follicles in the small intestine that serve as inductive sites for mucosal immunity. Here, B cells recognize microbial antigens presented by dendritic cells and undergo class-switch recombination, predominantly producing immunoglobulin A (IgA). The key roles of IgA include neutralizing pathogens and preventing the translocation of microbes across the mucosal barrier. Furthermore, the diverse microbial communities in the gut stimulate a broad repertoire of IgA, thereby ensuring a robust immune defense[73].

Th17 cells, a subset of CD4+ T cells, play a key role in mucosal defense against fungi and extracellular bacteria, promote barrier integrity, and produce interleukin-17 (IL-17) and IL-22. The gut microbiota has a strong influence on the differentiation and expansion of Th17 cells. However, an overabundance of Th17-promoting microbes, such as segmented filamentous bacteria (SFB), can lead to excessive inflammation and contribute to the development of autoimmune diseases. For instance, colonization of mice with SFB has been linked to increased Th17 cell activity and the onset of experimental autoimmune encephalomyelitis (EAE), a model for multiple sclerosis[74]. This demonstrates the delicate balance required in microbial communities to support immune function without precipitating harmful inflammatory responses.

Dysbiosis and Immune Dysregulation

Microbial dysbiosis refers to the disruption of the equilibrium between immune tolerance and activation, which can contribute to various immune-mediated diseases. This imbalance can manifest in numerous ways, affecting both local and systemic immune responses. Examples include the following pathologies:

Inflammatory Bowel Disease (IBD): Patients with IBD often exhibit reduced levels of SCFA-producing bacteria, such as *Faecalibacterium prausnitzii*, while showing increased populations of pro-inflammatory taxa, including *Escherichia coli*. This imbalance contributes to enhanced epithelial permeability and TLR signaling, which in turn fuels chronic inflammation within the gut[75]. The disruption of the microbial community and its effects on immune responses highlight the need for targeted interventions to restore microbial balance in IBD patients.

Allergy and Asthma: A significant reduction in microbial diversity during early life is associated with impaired Treg development and heightened Th2 responses, which can contribute to the development of allergic sensitization. Research indicates that exposure to diverse microbial environments in infancy, particularly those found in rural settings, is associated with lower rates of asthma and allergies[76]. This suggests that early microbial exposures may play a protective role against the development of allergic diseases.

Autoimmune Diseases: Dysbiosis has been implicated in the pathogenesis of several autoimmune diseases, such as type 1 diabetes (T1D) and rheumatoid arthritis (RA). In mouse models prone to type 1 diabetes (T1D), alterations in the microbiome precede disease onset and correlate with reduced gut barrier integrity and systemic immune activation[77]. This relationship underscores the potential of microbiome-targeted therapies in preventing or mitigating autoimmune conditions.

Infections: The depletion of beneficial commensal microbes through antibiotic use significantly reduces both microbial diversity and colonization resistance, allowing opportunistic pathogens such as *Clostridioides difficile* to proliferate. Restoring microbial diversity is essential for reestablishing colonization resistance and preventing disease[78].

Epilogue

The gut microbiome plays an integral role in the development, function, and tolerance of the immune system. Through continuous interactions with GALT, regulatory T cells, and both innate and adaptive immune responses, the microbiota effectively educates and calibrates the immune response. Dysbiosis, whether induced by antibiotics, dietary choices, or environmental factors, can disrupt this delicate balance, leading to an increased risk of various inflammatory, allergic, and autoimmune conditions. Therefore, restoring microbial balance through dietary interventions, probiotics, or more advanced therapeutic approaches holds significant promise for modulating the immune system and preventing disease.

Chapter 5

Impact of Food and Lifestyle Factors on the Microbiome

Introduction

The age-old adage "you are what you eat" gains scientific validation when examined through the lens of the gut microbiome. Our digestive tract harbors trillions of microorganisms—bacteria, viruses, fungi, and archaea—collectively known as the gut microbiota. These organisms are not passive residents; they actively interact with the food we consume, converting it into molecular messages that influence host metabolism, immune regulation, and even brain function. Food is thus more than mere sustenance—it acts as information that programs the gut ecosystem and, in turn, affects systemic health.

How Different Diets Affect Gut Flora

Assuming optimum hydration, fiber is arguably the most critical component for maintaining a healthy microbiome. Soluble fibers, such as those found in oats, apples, and beans, are fermented by gut bacteria into SCFAs, which are essential for various bodily functions. Insoluble fibers, derived from whole grains and vegetables, aid in maintaining digestive motility and fecal bulk. A lack of dietary fiber can force microbes to consume the host's mucus layer, potentially leading to increased gut permeability, commonly referred to as "leaky gut," and inflammation[79]. The importance of incorporating sufficient fiber into the diet is evident in a comparison of the relative microbiome profiles of individuals consuming a Mediterranean diet versus those consuming a Western-style diet.

The Mediterranean diet, which emphasizes the consumption of fruits, vegetables, whole grains, legumes, nuts, and olive oil, has been linked to a particularly favorable microbial profile, such as *Prevotella, Bifidobacterium*, and *Lactobacillus*. This diet not only boosts the abundance of SCFA-producing microbes but is also associated with lower levels of *Enterobacteriaceae*, a family of bacteria that can be potentially pathogenic. SCFAs, formed by the fermentation of dietary fibers in the colon, have been shown to play a crucial role in supporting gut barrier integrity and exerting anti-inflammatory effects[40]. Adherence to a Mediterranean-style diet for one year has been shown to result in improved microbial diversity and reduced markers of frailty and inflammation in older adults, showcasing the profound impact that dietary patterns can have on gut health[80].

Conversely, the Western diet, characterized by the consumption of ultra-processed foods (UPFs) that are often high in refined sugars, unhealthy fats, and artificial additives, can lead to overeating due to their hyperpalatable nature and content of chemicals that manipulate the brain's reward system, resulting in addictive-like behaviors. By promoting dysbiosis, excessive consumption of these foods can lead to inflammation, leaky gut syndrome, and metabolic dysfunction[81]. From a microbiome perspective, ultra-processed foods have been shown to decrease the abundance of SCFA-producing microbes while promoting pathogenic bacteria, such as *Escherichia coli* and *Clostridium difficile*. A 2014 study demonstrated that consuming an animal-based diet—rich in meat, cheese, and eggs—for just a few days caused a notable increase in bile-tolerant bacteria, such as *Alistipes*, *Bilophila*, and *Bacteroides,* while simultaneously reducing the abundance of fiber-fermenting bacteria, including *Roseburia* and Eubacterium rectale[82].

A high sugar intake, likewise, has been shown to promote the overgrowth of pathogenic microbes such as Candida and can increase levels of pro-inflammatory *Proteobacteria*. Furthermore, artificial sweeteners like saccharin, aspartame, and sucralose have been found to disrupt microbial composition and impair glucose tolerance by disturbing the delicate balance of gut microbes. This highlights the importance of moderating sugar and sweetener intake for maintaining gut health.

Research in 2015, using animal models, showed that food emulsifiers, such as polysorbate-80 and carboxymethyl-cellulose, can disrupt the mucus barrier, promote bacterial encroachment, and trigger low-grade inflammation and metabolic syndrome.

On the other end of the spectrum, ketogenic diets, which are high in fat and very low in carbohydrates, can alter the gut microbiome in both positive and negative ways. While ketogenic diets may provide benefits for individuals who have epilepsy or certain neurological conditions, prolonged use without adequate fiber can lead to a decrease in microbial diversity and reduced SCFA production[83]. This highlights the need for a balanced approach to dietary choices, especially when considering the long-term effects on gut health.

Likewise, high-protein, low-fiber diets, commonly adopted by athletes and bodybuilders, may also shift the microbiota toward proteolytic fermentation. This shift can lead to the production of potentially harmful metabolites, such as ammonia, phenols, and hydrogen sulfide, particularly when there is insufficient fiber intake to balance the fermentation processes[84].

Lifestyle Factors Influencing Gut Health

Additionally, modern lifestyles often subject individuals to psychological stress, sleep disruption, and exposure to environmental pollutants, all of which can negatively impact the gut microbiota. Chronic psychological stress can lead to dysbiosis through its influence on the gut-brain axis, resulting in increased intestinal permeability, often referred to as "leaky gut." This imbalance can manifest in symptoms such as irritable bowel syndrome (IBS), anxiety, and fatigue. Employing stress-reduction techniques, such as mindfulness and meditation, may help individuals maintain microbial balance and overall gut health[39].

Poor sleep can disrupt circadian rhythms that are crucial for regulating microbial activity in the gut. Disruptions in sleep and circadian cycles can lead to a decrease in microbial diversity, which is associated with metabolic dysfunctions such as insulin resistance and weight gain[85].

Engaging in regular exercise has been linked to increased microbial diversity and an enrichment of health-promoting bacterial species within the gut. Active individuals often exhibit higher levels of short-chain fatty acids, which contribute positively to gut health[86].

Furthermore, environmental pollutants—whether from heavy metals, pesticides, or airborne toxins—can also disrupt the gut ecosystem. These harmful substances may diminish beneficial bacteria, stimulate pro-inflammatory strains, and compromise the gut barrier[87]. The rising presence of microplastics in the food chain adds another layer of complexity, serving as vectors for harmful chemicals and microbes that can adversely impact gut health.

While modern conveniences, such as antibiotics and sanitized environments, have improved hygiene and survival, they have also disrupted the microbial ecosystem that co-evolved with humans. Reduced exposure to diverse environmental microbes may contribute to the rise of autoimmune and allergic diseases in developed countries[88].

Epilogue

Modern life presents a paradox: although we enjoy longer lives and cleaner environments, we are also more susceptible to diseases linked to microbial imbalance. From antibiotic use to the effects of artificial lighting, every choice and exposure influences our internal ecosystems. Understanding these interactions is crucial for restoring and maintaining microbiome health in the 21st century. By making informed decisions about diet, lifestyle, and environmental exposures, individuals can take proactive steps to enhance gut health, which in turn supports overall well-being.

Chapter 6

Signs of a Healthy (or Unhealthy) Gut Microbiome

Introduction

The human gastrointestinal system serves not only as a digestive organ but also as a sophisticated ecosystem populated by trillions of microbes known as the gut microbiota. This active community has a significant impact on human health, affecting metabolism, immunity, mood, and cognitive function. A balanced gut microbiota fosters health and resilience, whereas disruptions—termed dysbiosis—can lead to widespread effects. Recognizing the indicators of a healthy or unhealthy gut microbiome enables individuals to make informed lifestyle decisions for better well-being.

What a Healthy Gut Looks Like
from a Microbiome Perspective

Despite tens of thousands of studies and substantial global efforts to characterize the human gut microbiota, science has yet to define what constitutes a "healthy microbiome" or provide specific guidelines on how to modify it to achieve desired health outcomes. This can only be achieved over time through rigorous, standardized human intervention studies where researchers examine the causal links between diet, the microbiome, and health outcomes. While no single microbial profile currently defines health universally, researchers have identified consistent features in balanced microbiomes. These include a balanced ratio of beneficial bacteria to opportunistic species, microbial diversity, efficient SCFA production, increased capacity for vitamin and neurotransmitter synthesis, and the presence of a robust epithelial mucus layer. Of these parameters, the two most reliable quantitative metrics for assessing the health of the microbiome are the Gut Microbiome Health Index (GMHI) and the Gut Microbiome Wellness Index (GMW2).

The Gut Microbiome Health Index (GMHI) is calculated as the ratio of the relative abundances of health-associated species to disease-associated/opportunistic species[89]. Similarly, the updated Gut Microbiome Wellness Index (GMW2) utilizes a logarithmic ratio of beneficial to opportunistic taxa to predict overall health status[90].

A healthy gut is protected by a robust mucus layer that functions as a physical barrier against harmful pathogens and toxins. The integrity of this barrier is bolstered by beneficial microbes and short-chain fatty acids (SCFAs) that these microbes produce. When this barrier is compromised, it can lead to microbial translocation into the bloodstream, triggering systemic inflammation and significantly increasing the risk of developing chronic diseases. Maintaining this delicate balance is crucial for overall health, as disruptions can lead to a cascade of health issues beyond the gastrointestinal tract. Therefore, understanding the functions of gut microbiota is essential for promoting long-term health and preventing disease.

A diverse gut microbiota is also a hallmark of health. Diversity ensures ecological resilience, meaning that the gut can resist and recover from disturbances such as infections or dietary changes. Lower microbial diversity has been linked with inflammatory bowel disease, obesity, and depression[91].

Beneficial microbes, such as *Bifidobacteria, Lactobacilli,* and *Faecalibacterium prausnitzii,* ferment dietary fibers into short-chain fatty acids (SCFAs), including butyrate, acetate, and propionate. These metabolites fuel colon cells, help to maintain mucosal integrity, modulate the immune system, and inhibit pathogens. SCFA deficiencies are common in dysbiosis and correlate with inflammatory diseases.

Many gut bacteria synthesize essential nutrients, such as vitamin K2, biotin, and vitamin B12, as well as neurotransmitters like serotonin and dopamine precursors. These nutraceuticals make a significant contribution to health and well-being. Animal model research studies have demonstrated that when the gut microbiome is disrupted, alterations in brain chemistry and stress responses occur, further confirming the gut's role in neurological health[92].

Characteristics of an Unhealthy Gut from a Microbiome Perspective

Consuming a low-fiber, ultra-processed food diet over a prolonged period results in the thinning of the mucosal layer surrounding the gut epithelium, a reduced ratio of beneficial to pathogenic microorganisms, and a decrease in microbiota richness and diversity. Such gut dysbiosis can arise from a variety of internal and external factors, including diet, stress, environmental toxins, infections, and the excessive use of pharmaceuticals, such as antibiotics. A dysbiotic gut can compromise immune surveillance. Belkaid and Hand[66] explained that maintaining microbial balance is crucial for educating the immune system to differentiate between harmful and harmless entities, with disruptions potentially causing increased vulnerability to infections, immunodeficiency, and autoimmune conditions. Guinane and Cotter[93] observed that reduced microbial diversity and the prevalence of opportunistic pathogens can disrupt normal digestive functions, resulting in discomfort and malabsorption. Additionally, microbial byproducts such as lipopolysaccharides (LPS) can trigger systemic inflammation, leading to fatigue[94].

Small Intestinal Bacterial Overgrowth (SIBO) and Small Intestinal Fungal Overgrowth (SIFO) are gastrointestinal disorders characterized by an excessive growth of bacteria and fungi in the small intestine, where bacterial and fungal concentrations are commonly relatively low compared to the colon[95]. In these conditions, bacteria and or fungi that typically reside in the large intestine migrate into or proliferate excessively within the small intestine. Several dysfunctional conditions often rooted in or affecting the colon or downstream bowel can contribute to these pathologies. These can include impaired motility resulting in transit delay, gut disruption following surgical intervention, immune or barrier dysfunction, changes in the gut environment due to a defective ileocecal valve, leading to a backwash of contents from the colon into the small intestine, and the long-term use of certain medications such as antibiotics and or proton pump inhibitors[96].

The regions of the small intestine that are most affected during SIBO and SIFO are the duodenum, jejunum, and ileum—the segments of the small intestine responsible for nutrient breakdown and absorption. Because the small intestine is not designed to host large populations of bacteria or fungi, this overgrowth disrupts normal digestion and absorption, leading to symptoms such as bloating, abdominal pain, diarrhea, constipation, malabsorption, and nutrient deficiencies, particularly of vitamin B12, iron, and fat-soluble vitamins.

The secondary effects of gut microbiome disruption on the brain, endocrine system, immune system, and skin are well established.

Because the gut and brain maintain a close connection through the gut-brain axis, gut dysbiosis can manifest in some patients as anxiety, depression, and cognitive decline. For this reason, researchers are currently evaluating the potential of microbiome-targeted therapies for addressing psychiatric symptoms, substantiating what is already well known: that gut health is vital for mental wellness.

Likewise, skin issues, including acne, eczema, rosacea, and psoriasis, have been linked to the health of the gut. The gut-skin connection illustrates how inflammation and microbial metabolites can affect skin balance. Bowe and Logan[97] suggested that increased intestinal permeability, often referred to as "leaky gut," can permit inflammatory substances into the bloodstream, worsening skin conditions.

Food intolerances, which differ from allergies, can stem from microbial imbalance or a weakened gut lining. Impaired digestion may allow undigested food particles to enter the intestinal barrier, triggering immune responses. This has been confirmed in studies, which found higher intestinal permeability in individuals with food sensitivities and autoimmune disorders, underscoring the gut's role in developing oral tolerance[98].

Epilogue

By perceiving the gut as both a mirror and mediator of health, individuals and healthcare providers can leverage microbiome science to inform lifestyle and therapeutic choices. This understanding can result in more favorable outcomes in terms of health and disease prevention. As research continues to evolve, the integration of microbiome insights into healthcare practices will play a pivotal role in enhancing patient care and promoting sustainable health improvements. This holistic view encourages an initiative-taking approach to health, emphasizing the significance of the gut microbiome in achieving optimal wellness.

Chapter 7

Clinical Strategies and Tracking Tools to Maintain Gut Health

Introduction

Gut health has emerged as a cornerstone of overall well-being, playing a pivotal role in digestion, immunity, mood regulation, and the prevention of chronic diseases. Yet, it is far from a fixed attribute; gut health continuously responds to internal and external influences such as diet, stress, medication, and environmental exposures. Recognizing and responding to these changes requires a combination of clinical insight, self-awareness, and technological support. Through professional guidance, community engagement, and regular monitoring, individuals can successfully track and maintain their gut health using an array of strategies and tools.

The Role of Professional and Community Support

One of the most foundational steps in maintaining gut health is building a strong support system. Working with experienced healthcare practitioners—especially those specializing in functional or integrative medicine—can offer a comprehensive view of an individual's overall health landscape. These professionals approach gut health with a broader lens, considering not only gastrointestinal symptoms but also lifestyle, psychological well-being, and systemic health markers.

Registered dietitians and certified gut health coaches are equally crucial in this journey. They offer evidence-based nutritional advice and lifestyle interventions tailored to an individual's unique physiology and needs. Their guidance can be instrumental in creating sustainable, gut-friendly routines, including anti-inflammatory diets, elimination protocols, or the strategic use of probiotics and prebiotics.

In addition to professional guidance, community support through online forums and educational platforms enhances this journey. Reputable websites, such as **Wellness Mama, MindBodyGreen,** and **The Gut Health MD,** provide access to the latest research, actionable advice, and forums where individuals can share their experiences and tips. These communities foster a sense of belonging and accountability while serving as a rich resource for troubleshooting challenges and celebrating progress.

The Value of Microbiome Testing

Gut transit time is a critical, adjustable factor that affects the composition and function of the microbiome. It is defined as the time between eating a standardized muffin inoculated with a dye and the first appearance of this marker substance in the stool[99]. Clinically, this can be easily measured using the blue dye method, also known as the "blue poop challenge." The shorter the transit time, the healthier the gut microbiome, and the longer, the worse. Gut transit time acts as both a marker and a mediator of health, linking diet, microbial activity, and disease risk. Improving transit time through dietary and lifestyle changes is an effective way to support a resilient and beneficial gut microbiome. Research indicates that gut transit time is a more reliable indicator of gut microbiome function than traditional measures, such as stool consistency and frequency[100].

Direct-to-consumer businesses offering microbiome analysis based on a single stool sample are experiencing rapid growth in popularity. These tests should be approached with caution, as many factors can influence the interpretation of stool analysis results. Instead, clients should consult a functional medicine physician for guidance on proper stool sample collection procedures and interpreting the laboratory microbiome analysis results.

Comprehensive stool analyses — such as those from **Viome**, **Genova Diagnostics**, **Thryve**, and **Ombre** —

deliver detailed reports that highlight imbalances or deficiencies within the microbiome. These platforms often include personalized dietary and lifestyle recommendations, helping individuals identify specific foods to include or avoid. For example, one person may be advised to reduce sugar intake and increase consumption of polyphenol-rich foods to foster microbial diversity. At the same time, another may benefit from increasing the intake of fermentable fibers to enhance the production of short-chain fatty acids. This individualized approach empowers users to take precise and meaningful steps toward improved gut health.

Breath tests analyze gases such as hydrogen and methane, which are produced through the process of microbial fermentation. These tests help identify intolerances to sugars such as lactose, fructose, or sucrose. They are also used in diagnosing SIBO—a condition where excess bacteria grow in the small intestine, causing bloating, discomfort, and nutrient malabsorption. Breath testing is crucial for differentiating between Irritable Bowel Syndrome (IBS) and SIBO[101]. The FoodMarble Aire 2 portable device, which measures both hydrogen and methane in the patient's breath, is a valuable tool in helping physicians diagnose gastrointestinal problems.

Intestinal permeability tests assess whether the gut lining is allowing larger molecules than usual to pass into the bloodstream, a condition commonly referred to as leaky gut. This is typically evaluated by measuring the translocation of molecules, such as lactulose and mannitol, or markers like zonulin, which regulate tight junctions between epithelial cells[102].

Markers such as calprotectin (a sign of inflammation), indican, and hippurate (byproducts of microbial metabolism) provide indirect evidence of microbial imbalance and intestinal inflammation. Advanced tests can also measure circulating lipopolysaccharide (LPS) or microbial DNA, indicating translocation of gut microbes into systemic circulation.

Diagnostic testing not only validates the presence of gut dysfunction but also guides the selection of therapies, including dietary interventions, probiotics, antimicrobials, and lifestyle modifications.

Digital Tools for Self-Monitoring

Advancements in technology have transformed how people monitor and manage their gut health. One of the most accessible and insightful tools is keeping a food and symptom journal. This involves recording daily meals and noting any related symptoms such as bloating, fatigue, acne, or mood changes. Over time, these logs can reveal patterns and identify triggers, making it easier to eliminate irritants and build healthier habits.

Mobile apps like **Cara Care** and **mySymptoms Food Diary & Symptom Tracker** are explicitly designed for this purpose. These apps offer a user-friendly interface for logging meals, tracking symptoms, and generating reports that can be shared with healthcare providers. They can help identify food sensitivities or intolerances that may not be detected by lab tests, offering real-world data to guide dietary adjustments.

At the same time, more general nutrition and fitness apps, such as **MyFitnessPal** and **Cronometer**, offer detailed views of macro- and micronutrient intake. These platforms enable users to track fiber intake—a crucial component for supporting beneficial gut bacteria—as well as hydration, protein consumption, and overall calorie intake. Tracking these factors helps ensure dietary choices support gut health.

For those seeking a more personalized approach, advanced programs at **Zoe.com** combine microbiome testing with continuous glucose monitoring and food response assessments. **Zoe** uses this data to create personalized dietary advice tailored to an individual's unique biology and how it responds to different foods. By integrating real-time feedback with microbiome analysis, **Zoe** promotes long-term adherence to gut-friendly diets and raises awareness of how daily habits impact overall health.

Monthly Check-ins: Connecting Data and Personal Experience

While lab data and app-based tracking give helpful insights, subjective self-assessment remains a crucial part of monitoring gut health. Monthly wellness check-ins can provide a reflective space for individuals to assess their body's response to changes. These check-ins can include questions such as:

- Are your bowel movements becoming more regular?
- Has bloating, reflux, or abdominal discomfort decreased?
- Do you notice improved energy and mental clarity?
- Has your skin become clearer or less inflamed?
- Are you sleeping better or feeling less anxious?

Answering these questions each month can uncover trends that aren't immediately obvious through lab tests or digital trackers. For instance, improvements in skin or mood may occur before changes in biomarkers, highlighting the interconnected nature of the gut-brain and gut-skin axes. Tracking these subjective changes can confirm the success of interventions and help your doctor or a professional health coach guide you with ongoing adjustments to your diet, supplements, or lifestyle habits.

Building and Adjusting a Sustainable Gut Health Strategy

Maintaining gut health is an ongoing process that requires consistent effort, curiosity, and flexibility. The aim is not perfection but responsiveness—being able to recognize what is working, what needs adjustment, and when to seek further support. As people learn more about how their bodies respond to specific foods, stressors, and interventions, they become empowered to take control of their gut health. This process builds resilience, promotes lifelong learning, and improves overall well-being.

Epilogue

By perceiving the gut as both a mirror and mediator of health, individuals and healthcare providers can leverage microbiome science to inform lifestyle and therapeutic choices. By combining microbiome science, the expertise of healthcare providers, the use of modern tracking tools, and a strong network of support, individuals can navigate their health journeys with confidence and clarity. This holistic view encourages an initiative-taking approach to health, emphasizing the significance of the gut microbiome in achieving optimal wellness.

Chapter 8

Strategies Supporting a Healthy Gut Microbiome

Introduction

The human gut serves as a vital interface between the body and the external environment, housing approximately 10 trillion microorganisms. It serves as the body's largest immune organ and plays a central role in digestion, nutrient absorption, and the regulation of neuroendocrine communication. When gut function is disrupted—due to imbalances in the microbiome (dysbiosis), inflammation, or increased intestinal permeability—it can lead to a wide range of systemic symptoms, such as digestive discomfort, cognitive difficulties, and skin conditions. Therefore, supporting gut healing is not just about alleviating symptoms; it requires a comprehensive approach that includes restoring microbial balance, repairing the intestinal lining, and adopting long-term habits that support gut health.

Achieving and maintaining a healthy gut typically involves a multifaceted approach that includes proper hydration, a diet rich in fiber, polyphenols, and fermented foods, effective stress management, sufficient sleep, and the careful use of medications. Each of these strategies plays a unique role in restoring a healthy microbial community, which is essential for overall health and well-being. By focusing on these therapeutic strategies, individuals can take meaningful steps toward improving their gut health..

Hydration

Adequate hydration is essential for maintaining digestive health, as it facilitates smooth nutrient absorption and promotes regular bowel movements. Sufficient water intake is crucial for maintaining the integrity of the mucosal lining and promoting a balanced microbial environment[103].

Dietary Fiber

Recent advances in nutritional science have highlighted the pivotal role of sustained dietary patterns in shaping the gut microbiome over time. Rather than focusing solely on isolated nutrients or individual foods, emerging research emphasizes the cumulative effect of diverse, fiber-rich, and plant-forward diets in fostering a resilient microbial ecosystem. Diversity in dietary intake acts as a continuous ecological force, selecting for a wide range of beneficial microbial taxa that collectively support immune modulation, metabolic health, and gastrointestinal integrity. Research indicates that consuming more than 30 different types of plant-based foods, rich in dietary fiber, each week is correlated with increased microbial diversity and a greater abundance of beneficial species[104, 105].

Nutritionally, two broad categories of plant-derived carbohydrates can be identified in the food we eat[106]. The glycemic carbohydrates are those that are digested and absorbed in the small intestine. In contrast, those carbohydrates and lignin (a complex aromatic polymer) that are non-digestible in the small intestine and pass into the large intestine constitute what is known as "Dietary Fiber". Some dietary fibers are water-soluble (found in oats, apples, citrus fruits, and legumes) while others are water-insoluble (found in whole grains, nuts, beans, cauliflower, and green beans). By adding bulk to stool, dietary fiber plays a vital role in regulating bowel movements. The recommended adult daily intake of fiber from food is 25–30 grams/day[106, 107].

In addition, some dietary fibers, such as resistant starch, inulin, fructo-oligosaccharides (FOS), and galacto-oligosaccharides (GOS), collectively known as microbiota-accessible carbohydrates (MACs), serve a prebiotic role[108]. These fibers travel through the small intestine undigested and reach the colon, where they undergo fermentation by beneficial gut species, such as *Bifidobacteria* and *Lactobacilli*. On average, the gut microbiota produce 500-600 mmol of short-chain fatty acids (SCFAs) daily, with acetate, butyrate, and propionate being the most abundant[109] [110]. These SCFAs buffer the gut's redox potential[109], are essential energy sources for colonocytes, strengthen gut barrier function, modulate the immune system, and have anti-inflammatory properties. Including prebiotic-rich foods in the diet also offers systemic benefits such as increased satiety, improved blood sugar control, lower cholesterol levels, and a reduced risk of colorectal cancer[111]. In addition to food sources of prebiotics, commercial prebiotic supplements are also available. The synergistic use of a prebiotic-rich diet, combined with prebiotic supplements, can significantly enhance microbiome recovery following a dysbiosis.

The histogram in Figure 1 lists the 15 foods richest in prebiotic fiber and grouped by culinary class. Quantitative data showing the prebiotic content of a wide range of foodstuffs across five culinary categories is given in Appendix 1.

Although chicory root and Jerusalem artichoke stand out as the richest natural sources of inulin-type fructans, making them true "prebiotic champions," they represent only part of the picture. Other food groups make distinct and complementary contributions to the prebiotic landscape. For example, allium vegetables such as garlic, onions, and leeks, while more modest in total fiber, are disproportionately high in fructo-oligosaccharides (FOS) and inulin, earning them a strong reputation as gut-health powerhouses[112]. Similarly, cereals like barley, rye, and oats provide β-glucans and arabinoxylans, fibers that are both highly fermentable and associated with cholesterol-lowering benefits[113]. Legumes add further diversity, offering galacto-oligosaccharides (GOS) and resistant starch that selectively nourish *Bifidobacteria* and *Lactobacillus*[114]. Seeds such as psyllium, chia, and flax contribute mucilage-rich fibers; although less selective than inulin or FOS, they still support broad fermentative activity and overall gut health[115].

When considered together, these examples underscore the importance of dietary diversity rather than reliance on a single "superfood." By incorporating a variety of plants, fruits, legumes, cereals, and seeds — each delivering distinct prebiotic compounds — individuals provide their gut microbiota with a broader spectrum of substrates. This variety promotes cross-feeding between microbes, enhances microbiome stability, and supports broader metabolic and healthier outcomes than can be achieved through consumption of only the highest-content sources[108, 116, 117].

In terms of good culinary practice, established food preparation methods (pressure cooking, soaking, and fermentation) are recommended to reduce the lectin content in certain foods, as lectin can affect the gut microbiome and worsen symptoms in some diseases[118-120].

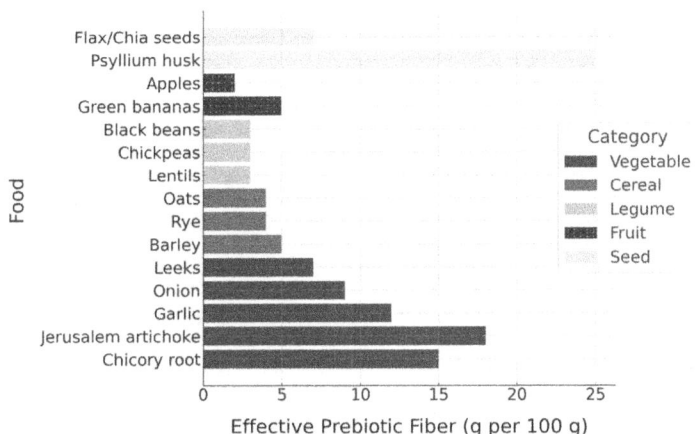

Figure.1 Top 15 Foods by Effective Prebiotic Fiber Content

Emerging evidence from preclinical research suggests that dietary interventions may be more effective than fecal microbiota transplantation (FMT) in restoring disrupted gut microbial communities. While FMT has been extensively studied as a method for reintroducing beneficial microorganisms, particularly in cases of recurrent *Clostridioides difficile* infection[121]—Its long-term efficacy in re-establishing a stable and diverse microbiome appears to be significantly influenced by the host's diet. Without a diet adequate in fiber and plant-derived polysaccharides, it seems that transplanted microbes fail to engraft or persist, highlighting the primacy of diet over one-time microbial interventions.

Food Polyphenols

In recent years, there has been growing scientific interest in the relationship between dietary polyphenols and the gut microbiome. Polyphenols have emerged as essential modulators of gut microbial composition and activity[122, 123].

Polyphenols are naturally occurring compounds found in a wide variety of plant-based foods. The richest sources include cloves, cocoa, dark chocolate (78% min. cocoa), green tea, berries, walnuts, and red onions (Table 1). The polyphenol content of other foods can be found in the book "Food For Life"[124].

Polyphenols are not fully absorbed in the small intestine; up to 90–95% reach the colon, where gut microbiota metabolize them into smaller bioactive compounds[125]. This biotransformation is mutually beneficial. While microbes help convert polyphenols into forms that are easier for the body to absorb, polyphenols can also inhibit the growth of harmful bacteria, such as *Clostridium perfringens* and *Escherichia coli*, while selectively promoting the development of beneficial gut bacteria, particularly those belonging to the *Bifidobacterium* and *Lactobacillus* genera[126] [127]. Specific polyphenols, including flavonoids (e.g., quercetin and catechins), stilbenes (e.g., resveratrol), and phenolic acids (e.g., caffeic acid), have been shown to positively impact microbial diversity and abundance.

Table 1
Top Ten Polyphenol-Rich Foods

Rank	Food	Category	Main Polyphenols	Approx. Content (mg/100 g)
1	Cloves (ground)	Spice	Eugenol, flavonoids	15,000–16,000
2	Star anise	Spice	Flavonoids, phenolic acids	5,500–7,500
3	Cocoa powder (unsweetened)	Chocolate / Seed	Flavanols	3,400–3,800
4	Dark chocolate (70–85% cacao)	Chocolate	Flavanols	1,500–2,000
5	Black elderberries	Fruit	Anthocyanins, flavonols	1,300–1,500
6	Black chokeberries (aronia)	Fruit	Anthocyanins, proanthocyanidins	1,200–1,600
7	Walnuts	Nut / Seed	Ellagitannins, flavonoids	1,200–1,400
8	Blueberries	Fruit	Anthocyanins, flavonols	400–600
9	Red onions	Vegetable	Quercetin	300–400
10	Green tea (dry leaves)	Beverage	Catechins	100–150 per g dry leaves (~3–5 cups brewed = 200–300 mg)

For example, green tea catechins promote the growth of *Akkermansia muciniphila*, a bacterium associated with enhanced metabolic health and improved gut barrier function[128]. Likewise, resveratrol from red wine has been linked to increased levels of SCFA-producing bacteria and enhanced insulin sensitivity in animal studies[129].

Polyphenols are recognized for their antioxidant, anti-inflammatory, and cardioprotective effects[130, 131]. By lowering oxidative stress and inflammatory signals in the gut, polyphenols help maintain mucosal integrity and prevent harmful bacteria and endotoxins from entering the bloodstream.[132] This modulation of microbial balance supports maintaining intestinal homeostasis, thus lowering the risk of dysbiosis, a condition associated with diabetes, inflammatory bowel disease (IBD), and even mental health issues[132, 133].

Thus, regular intake of polyphenol-rich foods may not only support digestive health but also offer systemic benefits, emphasizing the importance of a plant-rich, diverse diet for overall well-being.

Probiotic Foods & Supplements

Probiotics are live microorganisms that, when administered in adequate amounts, confer specific health benefits to the host. Probiotics are categorized by genus, species, and strain, with common genera including *Lactobacillus*,

Bifidobacterium, Saccharomyces, Streptococcus, and *Bacillus.* Each strain exerts different effects on health, making it essential to consider the specific purpose of probiotic supplementation[134].

High-quality probiotic supplements typically contain at least twenty billion colony-forming units (CFU) from thirteen or more live strains. While these beneficial microbes may not permanently colonize the gut, they are known to confer a range of health benefits, including improved digestion, modulation of the immune system, increased resilience, and a balanced microbial ecosystem within the gut[135, 136].

Fermented food sources of probiotics are generally preferred over commercial supplements. Among probiotic-rich foods, kefir is frequently highlighted as a powerhouse due to its superior microbial diversity. Kefir grains contain both bacteria and yeasts in a polysaccharide matrix, resulting in a beverage that provides up to 30 different strains of microorganisms.[121] Consuming kefir can be beneficial for digestion, promoting regular bowel movements, alleviating gastrointestinal issues such as diarrhea, constipation, and IBS symptoms, aiding in the absorption of nutrients (like calcium), and enhancing immune function. Notably, kefir is about 99% lactose-free, making it suitable for individuals with lactose intolerance. Other commonly recommended probiotic foods that support enhanced microbial diversity include yogurt with live cultures, produced by fermenting milk with *Lactobacillus bulgaricus* and *Streptococcus thermophilus*. Natural yogurt can aid digestion and improve lactose tolerance[136]. Fermented cabbage dishes, such as kimchi and sauerkraut, are not only rich in lactic acid bacteria, including *Lactobacillus* plantarum and *Leuconostoc mesenteroides*, but also, due to their fiber content, these products serve a prebiotic role. Kombucha, a fermented tea that contains both yeast and bacteria, including *Acetobacter* and *Gluconobacter* species, is also beneficial. Tempeh, a fermented soybean product from Indonesia, is another excellent source, containing *Rhizopus fungi* and beneficial bacterial metabolites. Foods like kimchi, sauerkraut, and tempeh are considered both probiotic and prebiotic, as their fermentation process enriches them with live microbes. At the same time, their fiber content feeds the existing beneficial bacteria, providing dual support for gut health.[111] Regular consumption of fermented foods has been shown to significantly enhance microbiome diversity and reduce levels of inflammatory cytokines[137]. These foods also provide bioactive compounds that improve gut motility and bolster immune function.

When selecting probiotic supplements, it is crucial to ensure that these products have a documented safety profile. They should contain "live and active cultures" and be stored under refrigeration conditions. Pasteurization or exposure to high heat can destroy the beneficial microbes. Labels should specifically indicate the presence of probiotic strains or live cultures, and products should be free from added sugars and artificial preservatives to maximize their health benefits. The efficacy of probiotics has been shown to be at its highest when taken before or during a meal rich in fats[138].

Immuno-compromised or critically ill patients should seek specialist advice before taking commercial probiotic supplements. Likewise, it is recommended that individuals with damaged heart valves discontinue taking probiotics before undergoing dental or surgical procedures. It is also very important to be aware that probiotics can influence the absorption and metabolism of certain drugs, such as those used in the treatment of cardiovascular disease[139].

Despite their rising popularity, probiotic supplements are not without controversy. A landmark study in 2018 challenged the widely held assumption that multi-strain probiotics are universally beneficial after antibiotic treatment[140]. The researchers conducted both mouse and human studies, discovering that individuals who took a commercial probiotic supplement after antibiotic treatment experienced a delayed restoration of their indigenous microbiome. Additionally, they faced incomplete mucosal recovery compared to spontaneous recovery or recovery via autologous fecal microbiota transplantation (aFMT) from scientifically screened fecal donor sources. The study also noted altered host gene expression related to gut homeostasis.

These findings suggest that while commercial probiotic supplements can colonize the gut, they may hinder the reconstitution of the indigenous microbiome. The study emphasized that the effects of probiotics are highly individualized, indicating that interventions such as diet-based restoration or aFMT might be more effective and safer. This nuanced perspective highlights the complexity of gut microbiome interactions and raises important questions regarding the universal applicability of probiotic supplements. As research continues to progress, the personalization of probiotic strategies tailored to individual microbiomes will likely become a cornerstone of future dietary and medical practices.

Postbiotics

Postbiotics refer to the metabolic byproducts of microbial fermentation that exert various biological effects. These byproducts include SCFAs, antimicrobial peptides (bacteriocins, reuterin), exopolysaccharides, and vitamins such as vitamin K and B12, respectively. Research has shown that postbiotics can reduce inflammation, strengthen epithelial barriers, and influence host metabolism[141-143].

Other nutraceutical supplements

Supplements that can play a crucial role in supporting gut repair and boosting microbial resilience include L-glutamine, Zinc carnosine, digestive enzymes, and natural antimicrobial agents.

L-Glutamine, an amino acid that promotes enterocyte proliferation in the small intestine, regulates tight junction proteins, suppresses pro-inflammatory signaling pathways, and protects cells against apoptosis and cellular stresses during normal and pathological conditions[144].

Zinc carnosine supports mucosal integrity and helps to reduce gut inflammation.

Additionally, digestive enzyme supplements help break down macronutrients, thereby easing the burden on the gastrointestinal tract.

In instances of bacterial or fungal overgrowth, herbal antimicrobial agents such as oregano oil, berberine, and garlic extract are effective in reducing pathogenic species while preserving beneficial flora[121]. These compounds are often integrated into functional medicine protocols to mitigate the microbiome-disrupting effects of broad-spectrum antibiotics.

Licorice root (DGL) soothes mucosal inflammation and supports the repair processes. Additionally, slippery elm and marshmallow root create a mucilaginous barrier over the intestinal lining, offering relief from irritation.

Exercise

Engaging in regular physical activity can positively influence the microbiome, increasing both diversity and the abundance of beneficial taxa associated with optimal metabolic health. Research indicates that exercise can increase the *Bacteroidetes-to-Firmicutes* ratio, a change associated with improved metabolic health, lower rates of obesity, and greater gut diversity[145] [146]. Moderate-intensity activities such as brisk walking, yoga, or cycling not only stimulate intestinal motility but also help alleviate constipation. Consequently, incorporating regular exercise into one's lifestyle is essential for maintaining a healthy gut microbiome.

Stress Management

The gut-brain axis is a vital connection between mental health and digestive health, operating through neural, hormonal, and immune pathways. Chronic stress can disrupt gut microbial communities, leading to increased intestinal permeability, often referred to as "leaky gut," and promoting systemic inflammation. To mitigate these effects, it is helpful to incorporate calming practices into daily routines, such as spending time outdoors, practicing deep breathing, engaging in yoga, or using meditation and mindfulness techniques for 10-20 minutes each day. Taking breaks from digital devices can also help lower stress levels and support overall gut health.

Sleep Quality and the Microbiome

Quality sleep and the maintenance of circadian rhythms have a significant impact on gut microbial activity. Research indicates that sleep deprivation can alter the composition of the microbiota, reduce the production of short-chain fatty acids, and increase inflammation within the body. There is considerable ongoing research investigating how the gut microbiota composition can be modulated to improve sleep quality and resilience.

Several strategies have been shown to support gut and sleep health. One effective approach is promoting prebiotic and dietary support that encourages the growth of beneficial gut microbial taxa and the production of essential metabolites such as short-chain fatty acids and tryptophan derivatives. This can be achieved through a diet rich in fiber, including prebiotic foods like onions, garlic, oats, bananas, and asparagus, as well as resistant starch, and fermented foods such as yogurt, kefir, and kimchi. Including polyphenol-rich foods and dietary sources of tryptophan, such as eggs, poultry, and nuts, further enhances these benefits.

Another valuable strategy involves leveraging microbiome–transmitter pathways to increase microbial production or host availability of sleep-promoting metabolites, thereby supporting overall well-being and quality of rest. Recent research has demonstrated that some strains of *Lactobacillus reuteri* (NK33 in combination formulas, E9 in preclinical models) have the potential to improve sleep by affecting host melatonin production and by increasing other sleep-promoting compounds such as ergothioneine and GABA[147, 148 149, 150]. The significance of this research has been substantiated with the recent granting of a patent to the Swedish company BioGaia, in recognition of its *Lactobacillus reuteri* strains as producers of melatonin and adenosine for therapeutic use. In his book "Super Gut", Dr. William Davis emphasizes the importance of incorporating *Lactobacillus reuteri* into one's diet to boost the health of the small intestine, prevent SIBO, and enhance overall well-being[151]. He advocates for the consumption of *L. reuteri* yogurt, which can be made at home using his recommended method involving a specific starter culture and prebiotic fiber (inulin).

A third key strategy involves aligning lifestyle habits with circadian hygiene to improve both gut health and sleep quality. Combining microbiome-focused interventions with a consistent sleep–wake schedule, proper light exposure—bright during the day and dim in the evening—well-timed meals that avoid heavy late-night eating, effective stress management, and physical activity earlier in the day can significantly enhance microbial balance and promote more restorative sleep[152]. Ensuring seven to nine hours of quality rest each night is also crucial for maintaining stable gut function and boosting immune resilience.

A Clinical Protocol to Improve Sleep Quality

The goal of the protocol (Appendix 6) is to illustrate how to enhance sleep quality and resilience by restoring and modulating the gut microbiota, microbial metabolites, and gut-brain signaling.

Epilogue

In conclusion, the gut is not merely a digestive organ; it serves as a complex ecosystem that plays a central role in overall wellness. Implementing an action plan that prioritizes daily consumption of fiber-rich and fermented foods, along with regular physical activity, sufficient quality sleep, and stress management, can significantly influence gut health. These efforts contribute to creating an environment where trillions of beneficial microorganisms can thrive. A well-balanced microbiome supports various aspects of health, including sleep, energy levels, mood stability, digestion, and immune function. By fostering these conditions, individuals can enhance their resilience and long-term well-being.

Chapter 9

Culinary Medicine

A brief history of Culinary Medicine

Culinary Medicine electives first appeared in 1893, when the British Medical Journal invited medical students to take courses in "sick care and convalescent cookery" to enhance their practical knowledge essential for future patient care[153]. The first cooking and nutrition elective course in the United States was held in 2003 at SUNY Upstate Medical University in Syracuse, New York. In 2007, the inaugural conference titled "Healthy Kitchens, Healthy Lives – Caring for Our Patients and Ourselves" was organized by faculty from Harvard University. This event was the result of a collaboration between Harvard's School of Public Health and the renowned Culinary Institute of America. It featured culinary education through cooking demonstrations and interactive, hands-on workshops, along with informative nutrition classes[154].

In 2012, Tulane University established the first Culinary Medicine center at a U.S. medical school, later named the Goldring Center for Culinary Medicine (Appendix 1). This pioneering effort created a teaching kitchen within a medical school, establishing itself as a leader in the Culinary Medicine movement. This milestone marked the start of formal culinary and nutritional education in the American medical curriculum. Today, the movement has grown, with over 50 universities across the U.S. offering Culinary Medicine electives in their medical programs.

The movement has also expanded to include Europe and Latin America. In the United Kingdom, the Association for Nutrition established an Undergraduate Curriculum in Nutrition for newly qualified doctors, assuming this responsibility from the Academy of Medical Royal Colleges in 2018. This curriculum aims to provide medical students with the basic knowledge and skills in nutrition needed for their future practice.

An Overview of Culinary Medicine

Culinary medicine is an expanding, evidence-based discipline within the field of Lifestyle and Preventive Medicine. Unlike traditional medicine, it combines nutrition, psychology, and gastronomy to help healthcare providers and patients make better dietary choices. While it does not replace conventional medical treatments, it complements them by encouraging overall wellness and managing disease through a key modifiable factor: diet[155].

At the heart of culinary medicine is a close relationship with the gut microbiome, a complex ecosystem comprising trillions of microbes in the gastrointestinal tract. The microbiome plays a crucial role in regulating immune function, metabolism, nutrient absorption, and even mood and behavior. Understanding how specific foods influence the microbiome enables more personalized and effective dietary strategies. Together, culinary medicine and microbiome science form a strong partnership in pursuing holistic health. This approach marks a shift in how we view the role of food in medicine—no longer just as a source of nourishment, but as a healing tool.

The Goals of Culinary Medicine

Culinary medicine lies at the intersection of nutritional science and culinary practice. It translates complex scientific data into actionable steps for patients and healthcare providers, such as how to select, prepare, and enjoy foods that nourish the body. This field recognizes that food is not merely fuel, but also a source of information that influences biological processes at the cellular level. When dietary habits are tailored to support an individual's health profile, outcomes in chronic disease management can significantly improve.

Mindful eating, or fully focusing on the eating experience, is another core aspect of culinary medicine. It encourages individuals to slow down, chew thoroughly, and savor each bite, which can improve digestion and enhance meal satisfaction. Studies have shown that mindful eating can reduce overeating, improve metabolic markers, and foster a healthier relationship with food.

Behavioral strategies rooted in culinary medicine also address common barriers to healthy eating, such as time constraints, limited cooking skills, and budget concerns. Educational efforts focus on meal planning, smart grocery shopping, and batch cooking techniques that make nutritious meals more accessible and less intimidating.

Additionally, culinary medicine promotes culturally sensitive methodologies that honor and integrate traditional dietary practices. Rather than enforcing a one-size-fits-all diet, practitioners work with patients to adapt healthful principles to their individual preferences, cultural backgrounds, and lifestyle needs. This adaptability increases the likelihood of long-term dietary adherence and positive health outcomes.

Culinary medicine thrives on interdisciplinary collaboration. Physicians, dietitians, culinary professionals, public health advocates, and community organizers all contribute unique perspectives that enhance the effectiveness of dietary interventions. Together, they can design programs that address not only nutritional knowledge but also food preparation, accessibility, and cultural relevance.

Community initiatives play a vital role in this effort. Cooking classes offered through community centers and healthcare clinics can demystify healthy cooking and provide a hands-on experience. Urban gardens and farm-to-table programs increase access to fresh produce and reconnect individuals with the source of their food. Schools and workplaces can also serve as platforms for introducing concepts in culinary medicine, influencing behavior across generations and diverse environments.

Implementation in Healthcare Settings

Since dietary needs vary depending on individual conditions, no single diet suits everyone. Different health concerns require different meals, foods, and beverages. Culinary medicine provides practical tools to help prevent or manage disease conditions by promoting evidence-informed eating plans that are both enjoyable and sustainable. The following are a few examples of eating plans that culinary medicine teams can fashion to help patients with a range of different pathologies..

The Mediterranean diet is based on the traditional eating habits of people living in countries bordering the Mediterranean Sea—particularly Greece, Italy, and southern Spain. It emphasizes whole foods, including vegetables, fruits, legumes, nuts, and olive oil. Furthermore, it promotes a lifestyle centered on shared meals, enjoyment of food, and physical activity.

The DASH diet—short for Dietary Approaches to Stop Hypertension—is a flexible and balanced eating plan designed to help prevent or lower high blood pressure (hypertension). It was developed through research funded by the U.S. National Institutes of Health (NIH) and has been consistently ranked among the healthiest diets for heart and overall health. Nutritionally, it differs from the Mediterranean diet by limiting total fat and sodium intake and avoiding the consumption of red wine.

Similarly, a variety of customized dietary protocols are frequently utilized to identify food triggers and mitigate immune activation in the gut. Elimination diets, for instance, involve removing common allergens—such as gluten, dairy, eggs, soy, and corn—for a duration of three to six weeks, followed by a systematic reintroduction phase to pinpoint sensitivities. Research indicates that this method can be effective for managing both gastrointestinal symptoms and systemic issues, such as fatigue and joint pain[121].

The Gut & Psychology Syndrome (GAPS) diet is designed to support gut healing in individuals with neurodevelopmental disorders. This diet emphasizes nutrient-dense foods, bone broths, fermented vegetables, and healthy fats, all of which work together to repair the gut lining and replenish the microbiome[121].

The low-FODMAP diet, initially developed for individuals suffering from irritable bowel syndrome (IBS), restricts fermentable oligosaccharides, disaccharides, monosaccharides, and polyols—carbohydrates known to exacerbate bloating and discomfort. While this diet can be effective in the short term, it must be supervised to prevent long-term reductions in microbial diversity[156].

The Autoimmune Protocol (AIP), an extension of the Paleo diet, eliminates potential immune-reactive foods, including grains, legumes, nightshades, and seed-based oils. This approach has shown promise in treating autoimmune diseases such as Hashimoto's thyroiditis and inflammatory bowel disease by reducing gut inflammation and restoring immune tolerance[121].

Integration of Culinary Medicine into Medical Education Programs

Culinary medicine is slowly being integrated into medical education and clinical practice across various institutions worldwide. A small number of medical schools and allied organizations have introduced courses and certifications in culinary medicine to prepare healthcare providers for counseling patients on diet-related matters. These programs typically combine nutrition education with hands-on cooking classes, often led by a multidisciplinary team that includes dietitians, physicians, and chefs.

Training in culinary medicine equips clinicians with more than just nutritional knowledge; it enhances their ability to communicate effectively with patients about food and eating behaviors. For instance, a physician who understands how to cook healthy meals is better positioned to provide practical, relatable advice that resonates with patients' daily lives. This level of engagement fosters trust and encourages behavior change.

Patients, too, benefit from participating in culinary medicine workshops. Cooking classes tailored for individuals with specific conditions, such as hypertension or diabetes, help participants develop the skills and confidence to prepare meals aligned with their health goals. These community-based programs are particularly impactful in underserved areas, where access to nutrition education and food may be limited.

Culinary Medicine Resources and Tools

A growing body of practical resources in the field of culinary medicine is increasingly becoming available to both healthcare providers and patients. These include a repertoire of cookbooks and manuals (Appendix 2), culinary medicine-led cooking classes (Appendix 3), and a range of digital tools (Appendix 4).

Renowned medical professionals have collaborated with nutritionists and chefs to develop healthy recipes informed by the latest research on the microbiome. These healthy meal plans emphasize the use of whole ingredients, balanced macronutrients, and cooking techniques that preserve the nutritional value of foods. These evidence-based strategies turn the newest insights into gut health into practical dietary approaches that help prevent disease, aid recovery, and incorporate good nutrition into medical treatment.

Digital tools, such as mobile apps and virtual cooking classes, are also expanding access to culinary medicine. These platforms offer personalized meal planning, cooking tutorials, and dietary tracking, making it easier for individuals to apply medical nutrition advice in their kitchens.

Evidence and Outcomes of Training Programs in Culinary Medicine

Culinary medicine is increasingly supported by a robust and growing research literature demonstrating measurable benefits for both clinicians and patients. On the clinician side, participation in culinary medicine programs has been shown to increase confidence in discussing nutrition with patients, improve counseling skills, and lead to greater use of food-based interventions in clinical care.

A recent study of first-year medical students enrolled in a culinary medicine elective found that comfort in discussing food choices increased from about 29% before the course to over 90% afterward, familiarity with the Mediterranean diet rose from approximately 54% to 97% and understanding of the role of dietitians in the clinical setting also increased significantly[157]. Additionally, medical schools that have incorporated culinary medicine training into their core curriculum report that students not only enhance their knowledge of nutrition and self-efficacy but also start incorporating healthier eating behaviors into their own lives[158, 159].

On patient outcome measures, culinary medicine interventions have been associated with reduced HbA1c levels in patients with diabetes, better adherence to dietary patterns such as the Mediterranean or DASH diets, increased consumption of vegetables and dietary fiber, decreased reliance on ultra-processed foods, and, indirectly, enhanced microbiome diversity through diet shifts. While not every study measures all of these outcomes, a consistent pattern emerges in trials and pilot programs.

The University of Maryland study and similar research strongly support the conclusion that incorporating culinary medicine into medical training enhances students' preparedness and competency as future clinicians, ultimately equipping them to promote better patient health outcomes[159].

Epilogue

Culinary medicine represents a transformative approach to health that combines food, science, and behavior within a holistic framework. By acknowledging the central role of diet in both the prevention and treatment of disease, and by equipping individuals with the knowledge and skills to prepare health-promoting meals, culinary medicine empowers people to take charge of their well-being. It fosters a deeper connection to food, not just as fuel, but as a fundamental component of health, culture, and community.

As this field continues to evolve, it holds great promise in reshaping medical education, improving patient outcomes, and addressing some of the most pressing public health challenges of our time. By integrating the insights of microbiome research, mindful eating, and culinary skill-building, culinary medicine is poised to become a cornerstone of preventative and personalized care in the 21st century.

Chapter 10

Restoring Microbiome Health after Antibiotics

Taking Antibiotic Medication

Prescribed antibiotics should be taken exactly as directed by a healthcare professional, such as a medical doctor or pharmacist. It is essential to discuss the potential side effects of the prescribed antibiotics with your doctor. Some antibiotics can decrease the effectiveness of birth control and, due to a reduction in the normal vaginal protective microbiota (*Lactobacilli*), may cause vaginal yeast overgrowth in some women[160] [161].

Responsible Antibiotic Stewardship

Responsible antibiotic stewardship is crucial for preserving gut microbiome health and is one of the most effective strategies to mitigate unnecessary antibiotic use. Antibiotic stewardship programs are designed to optimize prescribing practices, ensuring that these powerful medications are utilized only when essential and with the correct choice, dosage, and duration. Public health initiatives that raise awareness about the implications of overusing antibiotics are necessary for curtailing the rise of antibiotic resistance and minimizing collateral damage to the microbiome[162].

The Impact of Antibiotics on the Gut Microbiome

Antibiotics are a cornerstone of modern medicine, having saved countless lives by effectively treating bacterial infections. However, while they target harmful pathogens, their effects on the broader community of bacteria within the human gut—collectively known as the gut microbiome—can be profound and enduring. The mammalian gut microbiome resembles a complex ecosystem, akin to a forest, where diverse microbial species interact to maintain stability and function. As outlined in previous chapters, the gut microbiome has a profound influence on human health, affecting not only digestion and immune function but also various aspects of mental well-being.

When antibiotics are administered, they disrupt this delicate balance, akin to a forest fire, that indiscriminately destroys both harmful and beneficial bacteria. This disruption leads to a reduction in microbial diversity, a shift in species composition, and impaired metabolic activity within the gut[163]. The resulting condition is known as antibiotic-induced dysbiosis (AID).

AID increases gut redox potential by reducing the numbers of anaerobic, fermentative, SCFA-producing microbes (e.g., *Bacteroides*, *Firmicutes)* while encouraging the expansion of oxygen-tolerant, opportunistic pathogens[164]. Furthermore, the simple carbon sources present in the Western high-sugar diet are quickly absorbed by the small intestine, limiting the carbon available for microbes in the large intestine. As these microbes compete for this limited carbon, they metabolize host-derived carbon from mucosal linings in the intestine[79]. This, in turn, increases gut inflammation and alters the microbiome structure by selecting bacteria that thrive in this inflammatory and aerobic environment, thereby reducing the ratio of beneficial to opportunistic microbiota. The depletion of SCFA-producing, beneficial gut bacteria severely compromises gut barrier function, increases intestinal permeability, and heightens susceptibility to infections and inflammation[165].

AID can manifest as a variety of gastrointestinal symptoms, including bloating, abdominal pain, diarrhea, constipation, and nausea. These symptoms arise because the depletion of beneficial bacteria, such as *Bifidobacteria* and *Lactobacilli*, compromises digestion and intestinal barrier integrity. One of the more severe consequences of dysbiosis is the increased vulnerability to opportunistic infections. *Clostridioides difficile* infection (CDI) exemplifies this, as the reduction of commensal bacteria following antibiotic treatment allows *C. difficile* to proliferate, potentially leading to life-threatening colitis[166].

The ramifications of antibiotic-induced dysbiosis extend beyond immediate gastrointestinal issues. Long-term alterations in the gut microbiome have been associated with various chronic conditions, including obesity, Type 2 diabetes, allergies, asthma, and even neurodevelopmental disorders such as autism[16]. Furthermore, the excessive use of antibiotics contributes to the emergence of antibiotic-resistant bacteria, which can persist in the gut and pose significant risks to public health by increasing the likelihood of infections that are difficult to treat[167]. Horizontal gene transfer among bacteria in the gut may facilitate the spread of resistance genes, thereby compounding this pressing issue.

The extent and duration of microbiome disruption can vary significantly based on the class of antibiotics used. A 2018 study revealed that even a single course of broad-spectrum antibiotics can dramatically alter gut microbiota composition in healthy individuals, with some microbial species failing to recover within six months[168]. Another longitudinal study highlighted that antibiotics such as macrolides and lacosamide, which exhibit vigorous anti-anaerobic activity, caused changes in the microbiome that persisted for up to four years post-treatment[169]. Individual factors, such as age, diet, prior microbiome composition, and environmental exposures, also influence the degree of microbiome damage. Notably, younger individuals tend to recover more rapidly than older adults, most likely due to differences in microbial resilience and diversity[170].

Studies Supporting Diet as a Tool for Microbiome Recovery

Among the various strategies proposed to support microbiome restoration, diet emerges as a foundational and modifiable factor that plays a crucial role in post-antibiotic recovery. The dietary use of prebiotics, polyphenols, and postbiotics has been discussed in detail in an earlier chapter.

A pivotal study, published in Nature this year, utilized a mouse model to investigate how dietary patterns impact the recovery of gut microbiota following antibiotic exposure[171]. In this study, mice were divided into two groups; one group was fed a high-fat, low-fiber "Western-style" diet, while a second group was given a high-fiber "Mediterranean-style" diet. The study demonstrated dramatically different outcomes in the recovery of the respective mouse microbiomes between the two dietary regimens.

The mice fed a "Western diet" showed both aggravation and poor recovery of their microbiome. A "Western" diet does not provide the necessary fermentable substrates, particularly complex plant polysaccharides (Microbiota Accessible Carbohydrates, (MACs)), that are vital for nourishing beneficial microbial taxa such as *Bifidobacteria* and *Faecalibacteria*[172]. Such a nutrient-poor environment frequently leads to the overgrowth of opportunistic species that can monopolize the available limited resources, thereby outcompeting other beneficial microbes that are essential for a full recovery. Consequently, the microbiome remains trapped in a state of dysbiosis, characterized by reduced diversity and resilience. This dysbiosis can predispose the host to a range of health issues, including inflammation, metabolic dysfunction, impaired immune regulation, and increased susceptibility to infections.

In stark contrast, mice that were fed the "Mediterranean style" diet exhibited a rapid and robust recovery of their microbiome. This high-fiber, MAC-rich diet was effective in facilitating the production of short-chain fatty acids (SCFAs) and other microbial metabolites, which create an optimal environment for microbial repopulation. Such an environment encourages the flourishing of diverse microbial communities, which helps restore ecological balance and fortifies the intestinal barrier[40]. The results highlight the significant role that a diet rich in microbiota-accessible carbohydrates plays in the recovery process following antibiotic treatment.

Notably, the study showed that diet alone was both necessary and sufficient for microbiome recovery, even outperforming fecal microbiota transplantation (FMT). In mice on the Western diet, FMT had little effect; the transplanted microbes couldn't colonize or diversify due to the poor nutritional environment. This highlights a key point: microbial recovery is mainly limited by the dietary environment. The findings suggest that focusing on dietary improvements, rather than relying solely on FMT, could be a more effective approach for restoring gut health in patients where antibiotics haven't fully eliminated beneficial microbial colonies. However, when the gut microbiome has been seriously disturbed—such as after long-term antibiotic use—a doctor might recommend combining fecal microbiota transplantation with dietary therapy to restore the microbiome. Autologous fecal microbiota transplantation (aFMT) is preferred over traditional allogenic FMT because it lowers the risk of pathogen transmission.

Another group of researchers studied the effect of the prebiotic, galacto-oligosaccharides (GOS), on microbial recovery in rats during antibiotic treatment[173]. The rats treated with antibiotics exhibited a significant decline in beneficial *Bifidobacteria* and *Lactobacillus* populations. However, those given GOS along with antibiotics had notably higher counts of these bacteria by day five after treatment. By day 15, their levels nearly returned to normal, and by day 20, they even surpassed baseline values. Interestingly, rats that received GOS after antibiotic therapy also demonstrated improved microbial recovery compared to the control group. Still, this recovery was slower and less complete than in rats receiving GOS during treatment. The study also found that GOS reduced levels of *Escherichia coli*. This common antibiotic-resistant pathogen aligns with previous findings that GOS may act as an anti-adhesive agent, preventing the colonization of harmful bacteria[174]. The conclusion from this research is that using prebiotics, particularly GOS, during antibiotic therapy helps restore the microbiota and promotes faster recovery of *Bifidobacterium* and *Lactobacillus* species.

Similarly, a study of the prebiotic properties of green banana flour (GBF), showed that this resistant starch food ingredient accelerated the restoration of gut microbiota and intestinal barrier function in mice following antibiotic treatment[175].

Given their importance, probiotics have garnered increasing attention for their role in restoring gut health following antibiotic treatments[176]. Several studies and reviews suggest that probiotics can help prevent antibiotic-associated diarrhea (AAD). A meta-analysis by Hempel et al found that probiotics, especially *Lactobacillus rhamnosus GG* and *Saccharomyces boulardii*, significantly reduced the risk of AAD, particularly in children[177]. In addition to preventing AAD, probiotic strains can temporarily colonize the gut, helping to re-establish microbial diversity that may have been lost during antibiotic treatment. Furthermore, probiotics have been shown to enhance immune function by modulating cytokine production and increasing the activity of natural killer cells and T lymphocytes[178].

Several expert groups and systematic studies recommend using multi-strain, higher colony-forming unit (CFU) dose probiotics before, during, and after antibiotic treatment. This proactive approach is believed to provide protection against gut flora depletion and promote the rapid restoration of microbial balance[177]. It is generally recommended to allow 2–3 hours between taking an antibiotic dose and a probiotic, allowing sufficient time for antibiotic absorption while minimizing the potential impact of the antibiotic on the efficacy of the probiotic[179]. This adjunctive therapy approach requires careful monitoring by a functional medicine physician, for reasons already outlined in a previous chapter.

Public health recommendations based on experimental evidence suggest increasing the intake of minimally processed whole foods, especially fruits, vegetables, legumes, and whole grains. In particular, consuming foods high in dietary fiber, prebiotics, polyphenols, and probiotics is crucial for supporting the recovery of the microbiome. On the other hand, individuals should limit their intake of ultra-processed foods, added sugars, preservatives, artificial additives, and alcohol, as these have been shown to disrupt microbial diversity and function[180]. It is also recommended that grapefruit and the juice of this sour citrus fruit should be avoided during the taking of all medications, including antibiotics, as this fruit is known to interfere with drug metabolism, potentially leading to increased drug toxicity or reduced drug effectiveness[181].

Thus, the experimental data from research so far support the idea that diet can act as a prescriptive or "medicinal" tool for restoring gut health after antibiotic treatment. By promoting the regrowth of commensal microbes suppressed during antibiotic therapy, dietary interventions can help increase SCFA production, which is essential for intestinal health, while also preventing the overgrowth of opportunistic pathogens and multidrug-resistant organisms.

Other Supporting Factors

Beyond diet, prebiotics, and probiotics, maintaining proper hydration, managing stress, and engaging in moderate-intensity exercise are also considered critical for promoting gut health. Both physical and mental stress can have detrimental effects on gut health, potentially leading to a microbiome imbalance. Addressing these lifestyle factors can enhance the overall effectiveness of dietary and probiotic interventions, providing a holistic approach to gut health recovery. By integrating these practices into daily life, individuals can support their gut health and overall well-being.

Post-Antibiotic Recovery Protocols

A structured, multifaceted recovery protocol should be incorporated into post-antibiotic care to enhance patient outcomes, minimize the recurrence of infections, and support long-term microbial and immune health.

Post-antibiotic recovery protocol summaries for both doctors and patients are available in Appendices 6–7. Patients should consult their family doctor at all times before commencing any post-antibiotic recovery protocol.

Epilogue

It is clear that the recovery of the gut microbiome following antibiotic therapy heavily depends on the quality of the host's diet and the targeted use of prebiotics. Research consistently demonstrates that a Western-style diet impairs microbial resilience and slows recovery. In contrast, a Mediterranean-style diet, rich in plant-based fiber, fosters a robust and diverse microbial ecosystem. Furthermore, prebiotic and probiotic supplementation—especially during antibiotic therapy—can significantly accelerate the restoration of key bacterial groups and reduce the overgrowth of pathogenic organisms. These findings carry substantial implications for clinical practice and personal health decisions.

Dietary interventions are cost-effective, non-invasive, and accessible strategies that not only support microbiome health but also contribute to broader metabolic and immune benefits. As microbiome science advances, the integration of dietary, prebiotic, and probiotic-based therapies into standard post-antibiotic care protocols holds promise for improving health outcomes and reducing the risk of long-term dysbiosis.

Chapter 11

The Future of
Microbiome Science

Introduction

The future of microbiome science is set to revolutionize our understanding of health and disease. The human microbiome, a dynamic assemblage of trillions of microorganisms that primarily inhabit the gut, is increasingly recognized as a vital factor in regulating metabolism, immunity, and even brain function. As research accelerates, the potential for groundbreaking advancements in precision medicine, disease prevention, and therapeutic interventions becomes clearer. Innovative approaches such as fecal microbiota transplants (FMTs), personalized nutrition powered by artificial intelligence, and microbiome-based diagnostics are paving the way for a new era in healthcare. This rapidly evolving field promises to deepen our understanding of the intricate relationships between microbes and human health.

The Microbiome and Endocrine Disorders

The recognition of the microbiome as an endocrine organ carries significant implications for the treatment and management of various endocrine disorders. Conditions such as obesity and metabolic syndrome, type 2 diabetes, polycystic ovarian syndrome (PCOS), mood disorders, and thyroid dysfunction can potentially be influenced by the state of the microbiome. Emerging research is exploring microbiome-targeted interventions, including the use of prebiotics, probiotics, dietary fiber, and fecal microbiota transplantation, as adjunct therapies in managing these endocrine diseases. By harnessing the power of the microbiome, healthcare practitioners may develop novel strategies to improve patient outcomes and enhance metabolic health. This evolving understanding of the microbiome's role in endocrine regulation is paving the way for innovative approaches to address complex health challenges.

Fecal Microbiota Transplants (FMTs)

Fecal microbiota transplantation (FMT) is a therapeutic procedure that involves transferring processed stool from a healthy donor into the gastrointestinal tract of a patient to restore microbial equilibrium. Initially developed to treat recurrent *Clostridioides difficile* infections (CDI), FMT has shown impressive success rates, resolving recurrent cases with efficacy exceeding 90%[182]. Given CDI's notorious resistance to standard antibiotic treatments, FMT represents a potentially life-saving option for affected individuals. Encouraged by these promising results, researchers are now investigating the application of FMT for a diverse range of conditions beyond CDI, to understand its benefits in various gastrointestinal and systemic disorders.

Research into FMT's broader therapeutic potential is expanding into several medical conditions. Inflammatory Bowel Disease (IBD), which encompasses Crohn's disease and ulcerative colitis, is a key area of interest. Emerging studies suggest a link between microbial imbalances and IBD, with some clinical trials indicating that FMT may induce remission in specific patient subsets. Another condition, Irritable Bowel Syndrome (IBS), characterized by a range of gastrointestinal symptoms, has also shown potential for improvement through FMT, despite the multifactorial nature of its pathogenesis. Furthermore, preliminary trials in children with Autism Spectrum Disorders (ASD) have reported behavioral improvements post-FMT, suggesting a connection between gut health and neurodevelopmental outcomes[183]. Lastly, investigations into obesity and metabolic syndrome highlight the impact of transferring stool from lean donors to obese recipients, which has shown temporary metabolic improvements, including enhanced insulin sensitivity[63].

Despite its potential, FMT is not without challenges. Variability among donors can lead to unpredictable outcomes, and the long-term consequences of altering a recipient's microbiome remain largely unknown. Regulatory bodies, such as the U.S. Food and Drug Administration (FDA), oversee FMT as an investigational new drug for all indications except CDI, necessitating careful consideration of ethical and regulatory issues[184]. As researchers work to standardize procedures, enhance donor screening, and explore synthetic stool alternatives, the future of FMT could see improvements that further validate its use as a viable treatment option.

Use of Live Biotherapeutic Products (LBP)

Although FMT has advanced the clinical use of microbiota, collecting healthy donor stool that is rigorously tested for the absence of potentially pathogenic agents remains challenging. The use of live biotherapeutic products (LBPs), which consist of consortia of commensal bacterial isolates, has been proposed as an alternative to FMT for controlling infections due to their improved safety profile and promising preclinical and clinical results[185]. An experimental study in a clinical mouse model, where mice infected with vancomycin-resistant enterococci (VRE) showed remarkable recovery following the administration of a consortium of seven commensal bacteria, demonstrated this approach's potential[186]. By enhancing gut barrier integrity and promoting microbiota recovery, this LBP effectively disrupted VRE colonization in the gut. These LBPs could also be used against other gut pathogens linked to dysbiosis.

Personalized Nutrition and Microbiome Mapping

The rise of personalized nutrition, guided by gut microbial analysis, marks a significant advancement in microbiome science. With innovations in next-generation sequencing (NGS), metabolomics, and artificial intelligence, it is now possible to analyze individual microbiomes and predict physiological responses to various foods. Commercial platforms, such as **Viome, DayTwo**, and **Zoe**, collect stool samples to assess microbial composition and functional potential, producing personalized dietary recommendations that aim to stabilize postprandial blood glucose levels, reduce systemic inflammation, and improve digestion. A landmark study demonstrated that personalized nutritional plans based on gut microbiome analysis significantly outperformed generic dietary advice in managing glycemic responses, underscoring the importance of individualized nutrition[187].

Machine learning algorithms continually enhance dietary recommendations by incorporating real-time data from users, thereby fostering an adaptive nutrition model that evolves in tandem with changes in microbiome composition. This shift from a one-size-fits-all approach to a precision nutrition paradigm represents a transformative evolution in dietary science and public health. By leveraging advanced technology and individual microbiome data, personalized nutrition can provide tailored strategies to optimize health and well-being.

The Microbiome's Role in Precision Medicine

The integration of microbiome science into the framework of precision medicine is revolutionizing the field of healthcare. This approach aims to tailor medical treatment to individual characteristics, including genetics, environmental factors, and microbial profiles. The microbiome's role in influencing drug metabolism, immune response, and disease susceptibility is crucial for informing diagnostics, predicting treatment outcomes, and developing novel therapeutic strategies.

Microbial biomarkers are being identified for a range of diseases, offering the potential for early detection and personalized interventions. In neurodegenerative disorders like Alzheimer's and Parkinson's disease, dysbiosis has been implicated in neuroinflammatory pathways that contribute to disease progression[188]. Similarly, specific bacterial strains, such as *Fusobacterium nucleatum*, are associated with colorectal cancer, paving the way for non-invasive stool tests that could facilitate early detection of this life-threatening condition.

Treatment personalization is another critical application of microbiome profiling, which can guide therapy choices by predicting how patients will respond to treatment. Research has shown that specific gut bacteria correlate with improved outcomes in cancer immunotherapy. A pivotal study found that patients with a diverse and favorable microbiota exhibited better responses to immune checkpoint inhibitors, suggesting that microbial composition may serve as a predictive biomarker for therapeutic efficacy[189].

The development of microbiome-targeted therapies is gaining traction as the field of microbiome science evolves. These innovative approaches include the use of synbiotics, which combine probiotics and prebiotics to enhance gut health synergistically. Other advancements involve designer probiotics engineered for specific functions, such as modulating the immune system. Postbiotics, which comprise beneficial microbial metabolites such as short-chain fatty acids (SCFAs), exhibit both metabolic and anti-inflammatory effects. Additionally, CRISPR-engineered microbes are capable of regulating gene expression, degrading toxins, and fighting pathogens[188]. As the science matures, microbiome-informed therapies may soon become commonplace in managing metabolic diseases, autoimmune disorders, infections, and mental health conditions.

Epilogue

The gut microbiome is not merely an ancillary component of human biology; it has a powerful and dynamic influence on overall health and well-being. The integration of microbiome science into contemporary healthcare signifies the advent of a new era in precision medicine. As we explore fecal microbiota transplants, personalized nutrition, and microbial diagnostics, we are only beginning to scratch the surface of the potential that lies ahead. The convergence of advanced technologies, such as artificial intelligence, multi-omics approaches, and synthetic biology, will likely yield increasingly sophisticated interventions aimed at optimizing the microbiome for therapeutic benefits.

While the path forward presents numerous challenges—including the need for standardized interventions, ensuring patient safety, navigating ethical considerations, and providing clinician education—these obstacles are surmountable. As our understanding of the microbiome deepens, its central role in diagnosing, treating, and preventing disease will become increasingly apparent. In the coming years, the concept of "microbial medicine" may become as integral to healthcare as genomics, shaping the future of individualized care and holistic health.

Appendix 1

Sources and Types of Prebiotics Across 5 Culinary Categories

1. Top Legumes

Rank	Legume	Prebiotic Fiber Type	grams/100 g
1	Lentils	Resistant starch, GOS	4–5 g
2	Red kidney beans	Resistant starch, GOS	4–5 g
3	Black beans	Resistant starch, GOS	3–4 g
4	Chickpeas	Resistant starch, GOS	3–4 g
5	Navy beans	Resistant starch, GOS	3–4 g
6	Pinto beans	Resistant starch, GOS	3–4 g
7	Soybeans	GOS	2–3 g
8	Split peas	Resistant starch, GOS	2–3 g
9	White beans	Resistant starch, GOS	2–3 g
10	Mung beans	GOS	2–3 g

2. Top Vegetables

Rank	Vegetable	Prebiotic Fiber Type	grams/100 g
1	Chicory root	Inulin	35–47 g
2	Jerusalem artichoke	Inulin	16–20 g
3	Dandelion greens	Inulin	13–15 g
4	Garlic	Inulin, FOS	12–13 g
5	Leeks	Inulin, FOS	10–12 g
6	Onions	Inulin, FOS	8–10 g
7	Okra	Mucilage, Pectin, FOS	3-4 g
8	Asparagus	Inulin	2–3 g
9	Beetroot	Resistant starch, FOS	2–3 g
10	Artichoke (globe)	Inulin	2–3 g
11	Green peas	Resistant starch, GOS	2–3 g

3. Top Fruits

Rank	Fruit	Prebiotic Fiber Type	grams/100 g
1	Green banana	Resistant starch	3–5 g
2	Unripe plantain	Resistant starch	3–4 g
3	Grapefruit	Pectin	2–3 g
4	Apples (with skin)	Pectin	1–2 g
5	Pomegranate	Polyphenols, FOS	1–2 g
6	Kiwi	Pectin, Inulin	1-2 g
7	Blueberries	Polyphenols, Pectin	1-2 g
8	Nectarines, Peaches	Pectin, FOS	1-2 g
9	Watermelon	Pectin	0.5 -1 g

4. Top 10 Seeds

Rank	Seed	Main Prebiotic Fiber Types	grams/100g
1	Psyllium husk (seed coat)	Arabinoxylans, mucilage (highly fermentable, gel-forming)	80–85
2	Chia seeds	Mucilage polysaccharides, soluble gums	~34.4
3	Flaxseeds	Mucilage polysaccharides, lignans	~27.3
4	Hemp seeds (whole)	Insoluble fiber + soluble polysaccharides	~27
5	Poppy seeds	Insoluble fiber, mucilage	~19.5
6	Sesame seeds	Lignans, mucilage, hemicellulose	~11.8
7	Mustard seeds	Mucilage, soluble gums	~10
8	Sunflower seeds	Cellulose, hemicellulose, pectic polysaccharides	~8.6
9	Quinoa (pseudo-seed)	Saponins, arabinans, and some resistant starch	~7
10	Pumpkin seeds	Cellulose, hemicellulose, pectins	~6

5. Top 10 Cereals

Rank	Cereal (whole grain)	Main Prebiotic Fiber Types	grams/100g
1	Bulgur (cracked wheat)	Arabinoxylans, cellulose, fructans	~18
2	Barley	β-glucans, arabinoxylans, fructans	~17.3
3	Rye	Arabinoxylans, fructans, β-glucans	~15.1
4	Wheat (whole grain)	Arabinoxylans, fructans (inulin-type), cellulose	~12.2
5	Oats	β-glucans (major prebiotic), arabinoxylans	~10.6
6	Millet (pearl millet)	Arabinoxylans, hemicellulose, resistant starch	~8.5
7	Maize (corn, whole kernel)	Resistant starch, arabinoxylans	~7.3
8	Sorghum	Arabinoxylans, resistant starch	~6.3
9	Wild rice	Hemicellulose, cellulose, resistant starch	~6.2
10	Brown rice	Cellulose, hemicellulose, arabinoxylans (small)	~3.5

Appendix 2

Culinary Medicine Healthy Recipe Cookbooks

Super Gut: A Four-Week Plan to Reprogram Your Microbiome, Restore Health, and Lose Weight (2023) by William Davis, M.D. Balance Publishing (Hachettebook.com).

Metabolical Cookbook: Easy & Delicious Recipes Inspired by Dr. Lustig's Teachings and Essential Insights for Optimal Metabolic Health (2024) by Josh Leach. Independently published.

The Dr. Gundry's Diet Cookbook: 300+ Lectin-Free Recipes with a 60-Day Gut Reset Plan to Boost Energy, Improve Digestion, and Encourage…. Loss Based on a Proven Nutritional Approach (2025) by Agnes J Ellis. Independently Published.

The Doctor's Kitchen - Eat to Beat Illness: A Simple Way to Cook and Live the Healthiest, Happiest Life (2019) by Dr. Rupy Aujla. HarperCollins Publishers.

The How Not to Die Cookbook (2018) by Dr. Michael Greger. Pan Macmillan Publishers.

How to Eat to Beat Disease Cookbook: 75 Healthy Recipes to Protect Your Well-Being (2021) by Dr. William Li with Ginger Hultin. Callisto Publishing.

The Food for Life Cookbook: 100+ recipes created with Zoe (2024) by Dr. Tim Spector. Jonathan Cape Publishers.

Chef MD's Big Book of Culinary Medicine: A Food Lover's Road Map to Losing Weight, Preventing Disease, and Getting Really Healthy (2008) by John La Puma, MD, and Rebecca Powell Marx, Harmony / Rod Publishers.

Culinary Medicine (2025) by Cheryl Casey, Scott Going, Lauren McCullagh, & Melanie Hingle. University of Arizona Publisher.

Culinary Medicine for Spine and Joint Pain: An Evidence-Based Approach (2025) by Caroline Varlotta, Rebecca Maitin, Joseph E. Herrera, Ana Bracilovic, and Grant Cooper. Springer Publishers.

The Body Reset Diet Smoothies (2023) by Pippa Campbell. Published by Rock Point, an Imprint of Quarto Publishing Group.

Appendix 3

Training Resources For Healthcare Providers & Patients

Program	Provider	Website
Health Meets Food	Culinary Medicine Curriculum, Tulane University, USA	https://goldringcenter.tulane.edu/
Nutrition and Global Health Research and Training Program	Harvard T.H. Chan School of Public Health Nutrition Program, USA	https://hsph.harvard.edu/research/nutrition-and-global-health/
Nutrition Education	Dr. Andrew Weil, Arizona Center for Integrative Medicine, USA	https://www.drweil.com/diet-nutrition
Healthy Kitchens, Healthy Lives	The Culinary Institute of America, USA	www.healthykitchens.org
Nutrition Pillar of Lifestyle Medicine	American College of Lifestyle Medicine, USA	www.lifestylemedicine.org
Foundations of Clinical Nutrition & How to Cook	Culinary Medicine UK	www.culinarymedicineuk.org
Online Nutrition Course	The Nutrition Institute, Ireland, Canada, South Africa, New Zealand, Australia, United Kingdom, USA	https://www.thenutritioninstitute.com/ie/en/
Cultural Models for Healthy Eating	Oldways, USA	https://oldwayspt.org/blog/plants-common-ground-worldwide-food-pyramids/
Food As Medicine Everyday (FAME)	National University of Natural Medicine, USA	www.foodasmedicineinstitute.com
Teaching Culinary Education across Medical, School, and Corporate settings	Teaching Kitchen Collaborative, USA	https://teachingkitchens.org/member-list/

Appendix 4

Web Addresses for Health Monitoring Tools & Apps

N	Tool /App	Web address
1	Cara Care	https://cara.care/en/
2	Cronometer	https://cronometer.com
3	DayTwo	https://daytwo-personalized-nutrition-ios.soft112.com
4	Everfit	https://www.everfit.io
5	Foogal	https://foogal.com
6	Genova Diagnostics	https://www.gdx.net
7	GI-MAP	https://www.diagnosticsolutionslab.com
8	MyFitnessPal	https://www.myfitnesspal.com
9	MySymptoms	https://www.mysymptoms.net
10	Perfact	http://perfact.co
11	StoolOMX	https://www.diagnosticsolutionslab.com
12	Thryve	https://www.thryve.health
13	Viome	https://www.viome.com
14	Zoe	https://zoe.com

Appendix 5

Clinician Checklist: Microbiome-Targeted Sleep Support Protocol

Objective: Improve sleep quality through microbiome modulation

1. Baseline Assessment

- Collect sleep history using one of the standardized patient questionnaires, such as the Pittsburgh Sleep Quality Index (PSQI) / Insomnia Severity Index (ISI).
- Record GI symptoms and dietary habits.
- Consider stool microbiome testing only if recurrent insomnia + GI complaints.

2. Prebiotic & Dietary Support

- Encourage **prebiotic foods**: garlic, onions, oats, bananas, beans (Appendix 1).
- Add **fermented foods**: kefir, natural yogurt, sauerkraut, and kimchi.

- Promote **polyphenol-rich foods** (berries, green tea) (Table 1).
- Restrict refined sugar, ultra-processed foods, and alcohol.

3. Probiotic Strategy

- **Recommended strains:** *lactobacillus reuteri* (NK33, E9, or clinically tested strains).
- **Evidence:** Shown to modulate stress-related sleep disturbances, GABA pathways, and ergothioneine production.
- **Dosing:** Use validated commercial formulations; administer ≥2–3 hrs. apart from antibiotics if co-prescribed.
- **Duration:** 4–12 weeks, reassess at intervals.

4. Microbiome–Neurotransmitter Pathways

- Support **tryptophan metabolism** → serotonin/melatonin synthesis (eggs, poultry, nuts).
- Enhance **GABA activity** via specific probiotic strains.
- Promote **ergothioneine** production with *L. reuteri*.

5. Lifestyle Integration

- Regular sleep–wake cycles, light hygiene, timed meals.

- Moderate daily exercise, avoid intense activity late evening.
- Stress-reduction: mindfulness, CBT-I referral if persistent.

6. Monitoring & Safety

- Track sleep outcomes at 4 and 12 weeks.
- Document adherence and adverse events.
- Use caution in immuno-compromised or critically ill patients.

Appendix 6

Post-Antibiotic Recovery Protocol for Healthcare Professionals

1. Microbiome Restoration

- **Probiotics:** Initiate a multi-strain probiotic regimen (e.g., *Lactobacillus rhamnosus GG, Saccharomyces boulardii, Bifidobacterium longum*). Administer at least 2–3 hours apart from antibiotics to improve colonization efficacy. Continue for 2–4 weeks post-therapy.
- **Prebiotic intake:** Encourage dietary sources of inulin and resistant starch (e.g., garlic, onions, oats, bananas, legumes) to enhance beneficial bacterial proliferation.
- **Fermented foods:** Recommend daily inclusion of cultured products (e.g., yogurt with live cultures, kefir, sauerkraut, kimchi).

2. Nutritional Support

- **Dietary pattern:** Prescribe a balanced, anti-inflammatory diet high in fruits, vegetables, whole grains, lean proteins, and omega-3 fatty acids.
- **Hydration:** Ensure fluid intake of 30–35 mL/kg/day unless contraindicated.
- **Restrictions:** Counsel against high sugar, refined carbohydrate, processed food, and alcohol intake during recovery.

3. Immune Function Support

- **Micronutrient adequacy:** Assess and correct deficiencies in vitamin C, vitamin D, zinc, and selenium. Supplementation may be indicated if dietary intake is insufficient.
- **Lifestyle interventions:** Emphasize sleep hygiene (7–9 hours/night) and moderate physical activity for immune regulation.
- **Adjunctive therapies:** Consider immune-supportive botanicals (e.g., echinacea, astragalus) under clinician supervision.

4. Hepatic Support

- **Nutritional interventions:** Promote cruciferous vegetables, leafy greens, and beets to enhance detoxification pathways.
- **Avoidance strategies:** Advise limiting hepatotoxic substances (alcohol, high-fat processed foods, unnecessary pharmacological agents).
- **Herbal adjuncts:** Milk thistle or dandelion root tea may be considered if clinically appropriate.

5. Lifestyle and Monitoring

- **Physical activity:** Recommend low-to-moderate-intensity outdoor activity such as walking, with gradual progression.
- **Stress management:** Encourage mindfulness, meditation, or relaxation training (yoga) to reduce cortisol-related immune suppression.
- **Clinical follow-up:** Monitor gastrointestinal function, fatigue, and infection recurrence. Consider stool microbiome analysis in patients with recurrent dysbiosis.

Appendix 7

Patient Post Antibiotic Protocol to be Approved by your Doctor

1. Heal Your Gut

- **Take probiotics:** Use a good probiotic supplement for at least 2–4 weeks after finishing antibiotics. Yogurt, kefir, and sauerkraut are natural options.
- **Feed the good bacteria:** Eat foods like garlic, onions, oats, bananas, and beans. These "prebiotics" help healthy bacteria grow.
- **Add fermented foods:** Try kimchi, miso, or kombucha for extra support.

2. Eat to Recover

- **Eat nourishing foods:** Eat plenty of fruits, vegetables, fish, nuts, beans, and lean meats.
- **Drink plenty of water:** Staying hydrated helps your body flush out waste and heal.
- **Limit junk food:** Avoid too much sugar, processed snacks, and alcohol.

3. Support Your Immune System

- **Get your vitamins:** Vitamin C (citrus, peppers), vitamin D (sunlight, fortified foods), zinc (nuts, seeds), and selenium (Brazil nuts, seafood) help immunity.
- **Rest well:** Aim for 7–9 hours of sound sleep each night.
- **Gentle herbs:** Teas like echinacea or elderberry syrup may give extra support.

4. Be Kind to Your Liver

- **Eat liver-friendly foods:** Broccoli, kale, Brussels sprouts, and beets
- **Stay hydrated:** Try lemon water or herbal teas like dandelion or ginger.
- **Avoid overload:** Skip alcohol and limit ultra-processed foods.

5. Move and Relax

- **Stay active:** Go for walks, stretch, or do yoga. Movement helps digestion and boosts mood.
- **Manage stress:** Try meditation, breathing exercises, or journaling to stay calm and balanced.
- **Take it slow:** Don't rush back into heavy workouts until your energy returns.

6. Keep an Eye on Your Health

- **Listen to your body:** If you notice ongoing diarrhea, extreme tiredness, or frequent infections, talk to your doctor.
- **Follow up if needed:** Your healthcare provider may suggest tests or extra support if recovery is slow.

In short, after taking antibiotics, focus on rebuilding your gut, eating nourishing foods, getting enough rest, moving gently, and consulting your doctor if needed. These steps can help you feel stronger and healthier.

Information Sources

1. Marchesi, JR., Ravel, J. The vocabulary of microbiome research: a proposal. Microbiome. 2015;3(1):31.

2. Guarner, F. The gut microbiome: What do we know? Clin Liver Dis (Hoboken). 2015;5(4):86–90.

3. Daniel, H. Diet and the gut microbiome: from hype to hypothesis. Br J Nutr. 2020;124(6):521–30.

4. Sender, R., Fuchs, S., et al. Revised Estimates for the Number of Human and Bacterial Cells in the Body. PLoS Biol. 2016;14(8):e1002533.

5. Almeida, A., Mitchell, AL., et al. A new genomic blueprint of the human gut microbiota. Nature. 2019;568(7753):499–504.

6. Qin, J., Li, R., et al. A human gut microbial gene catalogue established by metagenomic sequencing. Nature. 2010;464(7285):59–65.

7. The Human Microbiome Project Consortium. Structure, function, and diversity of the healthy human microbiome. Nature. 2012;486(7402):207–14.

8. Davenport, ER., Sanders, JG., et al. The human microbiome in evolution. BMC Biology. 2017;15(1):127.

9. Domínguez-Bello, MG., Costello, EK., et al. Delivery mode shapes the acquisition and structure of the initial microbiota across multiple body habitats in newborns. Proc Natl Acad Sci U S A. 2010;107(26):11971–5.

10. Kennedy, KM., Plagemann, A., et al. Delivery mode, birth order, and sex impact neonatal microbial colonization. Gut Microbes. 2025;17(1):2491667.

11. Rothschild, D., Weissbrod, O., et al. Environment dominates over host genetics in shaping human gut microbiota. Nature. 2018;555(7695):210–5.

12. Turnbaugh, PJ., Hamady, M., et al. A core gut microbiome in obese and lean twins. Nature. 2009;457(7228):480–4.

13. Goodrich, JK., Waters, JL., et al. Human genetics shape the gut microbiome. Cell. 2014;159(4):789–99.

14. Peterson, J., Garges, S., et al. The NIH Human Microbiome Project. Genome Res. 2009;19(12):2317–23.

15. Turnbaugh, PJ., Ley, RE., et al. The human microbiome project. Nature. 2007;449(7164):804–10.

16. Cho, I., Blaser, MJ. The human microbiome: at the interface of health and disease. Nat Rev Genet. 2012;13(4):260–70.

17. Ramirez, J., Guarner, F., et al. Antibiotics as Major Disruptors of Gut Microbiota. Front Cell Infect Microbiol. 2020;10:572912.

18. Reyes, A., Haynes, M., et al. Viruses in the fecal microbiota of monozygotic twins and their mothers. Nature. 2010;466(7304):334–8.

19. Underhill, DM., Iliev, ID. The mycobiota: interactions between commensal fungi and the host immune system. Nat Rev Immunol. 2014;14(6):405–16.

20. Samuel, BS., Hansen, EE., et al. Genomic and metabolic adaptations of Methanobrevibacter smithii to the human gut. Proc Natl Acad Sci U S A. 2007;104(25):10643–8.

21. Arrieta, MC., Stiemsma, LT., et al. The intestinal microbiome in early life: health and disease. Front Immunol. 2014;5:427.

22. Bäckhed, F., Roswall, J., et al. Dynamics and Stabilization of the Human Gut Microbiome during the First Year of Life. Cell Host Microbe. 2015;17(5):690–703.

23. Harmsen, HJ., Wildeboer-Veloo, AC., et al. Analysis of intestinal flora development in breast-fed and formula-fed infants by using molecular identification and detection methods. J Pediatr Gastroenter. Nutr. 2000;30(1):61–7.

24. Martin, R., Nauta, AJ., et al. Early life: gut microbiota and immune development in infancy. Benef Microbes. 2010;1(4):367–82.

25. Scholtens, PA., Oozeer, R., et al. The early settlers: intestinal microbiology in early life. Annu Rev Food Sci Technol. 2012;3:425–47.

26. Orrhage, K., Nord, CE. Factors controlling the bacterial colonization of the intestine in breastfed infants. Acta Paediatr Suppl. 1999;88(430):47–57.

27. Ballard, O., Morrow, AL. Human milk composition: nutrients and bioactive factors. Pediatr Clin North Am. 2013;60(1):49–74.

28. Zivkovic, AM., German, JB., et al. Human Milk Glycobiome and Its Impact on the Infant Gastroint. Microbiota. Proc Natl Acad Sci. 2011;108 (Suppl 1):4653–8.

29. Bode, L. Human milk oligosaccharides: every baby needs a sugar mama. Glycobiology. 2012;22(9):1147–62.

30. Jost, T, Lacroix C., et al. Assessment of bacterial diversity in breast milk using culture-dependent and culture-independent approaches. Br J Nutr. 2013;110(7):1253–62.

31. Pannaraj, PS., Li, F., et al. Association Between Breast Milk Bacterial Communities and Establishment and Development of the Infant Gut Microbiome. JAMA Pediatr. 2017;171(7):647–54.

32. Claesson, MJ., Jeffery, IB., et al. Gut microbiota composition correlates with diet and health in the elderly. Nature. 2012;488(7410):178–84.

33. Wilmanski, T., Diener, C., et al. The gut microbiome pattern reflects healthy aging and predicts survival in humans. Nat Metab. 2021;3(2):274–86.

34. Biagi, E., Franceschi, C., et al. Gut Microbiota and Extreme Longevity. Curr Biol. 2016;26(11):1480–5.

35. Lozada-Martinez, ID., Lozada-Martinez, LM., et al. Gut microbiota in centenarians: A potential metabolic and aging regulator in the study of extreme longevity. Aging Med (Milton). 2024;7(3):406–13.

36. Gilbert, JA., Blaser, MJ., et al. Current understanding of the human microbiome. Nat Med. 2018;24(4):392–400.

37. Cryan, JF., Dinan, TG. Mind-altering microorganisms: the impact of the gut microbiota on brain and behaviour. Nat Rev Neurosci. 2012;13(10):701–12.

38. Clarke, G., Grenham, S., et al. The microbiome-gut-brain axis during early life regulates the hippocampal serotonergic system in a sex-dependent manner. Mol Psychiatry. 2013;18(6):666–73.

39. Foster, JA., Rinaman, L., et al. Stress & the gut-brain axis: Regulation by the microbiome. Neurobiol Stress. 2017;7:124–36.

40. Koh, A., De Vadder, F., et al. From Dietary Fiber to Host Physiology: Short-Chain Fatty Acids as Key Bacterial Metabolites. Cell. 2016;165(6):1332–45.

41. Canfora, EE., Jocken, JW. Short-chain fatty acids in control of body weight and insulin sensitivity. Nat Rev Endocrinol. 2015;11(10):577–91.

42. Brown, AJ., Goldsworthy, SM., et al. The Orphan G protein-coupled receptors GPR41 and GPR43 are activated by propionate and other short chain carboxylic acids. J Biol Chem. 2003;278(13):11312–9.

43. Silva, YP., Bernardi, A., et al. The Role of Short-Chain Fatty Acids From Gut Microbiota in Gut-Brain Communication. Front Endocrinol (Lausanne). 2020;11:25.

44. Yano, JM., Yu, K., et al. Indigenous bacteria from the gut microbiota regulate host serotonin biosynthesis. Cell. 2015;161(2):264–76.

45. O'Mahony, SM., Clarke, G., et al. Serotonin, tryptophan metabolism and the brain-gut-microbiome axis. Behav Brain Res. 2015;277:32–48.

46. Strandwitz, P. Neurotransmitter modulation by the gut microbiota. Brain Res. 2018;1693(Pt B):128–33.

47. Dinan, TG., Cryan, JF. The Microbiome-Gut-Brain Axis in Health and Disease. Gastroenterol Clin North Am. 2017;46(1):77–89.

48. Carabotti, M., Scirocco, A., et al. The gut-brain axis: interactions between enteric microbiota, central and enteric nervous systems. Ann Gastroenterol. 2015;28(2):203–9.

49. Bonaz, B., Bazin, T. The Vagus Nerve at the Interface of the Microbiota-Gut-Brain Axis. Front Neurosci. 2018;12:49.

50. Gershon, MD., Tack, J. The serotonin signaling system: from basic understanding to drug development for functional GI disorders. Gastroenterology. 2007;132(1):397–414.

51. Dinan, TG., Cryan JF. Gut instincts: microbiota as a key regulator of brain development, aging, and neurodegeneration. J Physiol. 2017;595(2):489–503.

52. Kang, DW., Adams JB., et al. Microbiota Transfer Therapy alters gut ecosystem and improves gastrointestinal and autism symptoms: an open-label study. Microbiome. 2017;5(1):10.

53. Möhle, L., Mattei, D., et al. Ly6C(hi) Monocytes Provide a Link between Antibiotic-Induced Changes in Gut Microbiota and Adult Hippocampal Neurogenesis. Cell Rep. 2016;15(9):1945–56.

54. Sudo, N., Chida, Y., et al. Postnatal microbial colonization programs the hypothalamic-pituitary-adrenal system for stress response in mice. J Physiol. 2004;558(Pt 1):263–75.

55. Trompette, A., Gollwitzer, E.S., et al. The gut microbiota's metabolism of dietary fiber influences both allergic airway disease and hematopoiesis. Nature Medicine. 2014;20(2):159 – 66.

56. Rasmussen, TS., Mentzel, CMJ., et al. The gut microbiome in asthma, allergy, and airway disease. Respiratory Research. 2020;21(1).

57. Xu, B., Wang, D., et al. Acupuncture regulates gut microbiota: A systematic review and meta-analysis. Frontiers in Microbiology. 2024;15.

58. Liu, Y., Zhu, C., et al. Effect and mechanism of acupuncture on the gut-lung axis in patients with chronic obstructive pulmonary disease. Medicine. 2025;104(5).

59. Sayin, SI., Wahlström, A., et al. Gut microbiota regulates bile acid metabolism by reducing the levels of tauro-beta-muricholic acid, a naturally occurring FXR antagonist. Cell Metab. 2013;17(2):225–35.

60. Ridlon, JM., Kang, DJ. Bile salt biotransformations by human intestinal bacteria. J Lipid Res. 2006;47(2):241–59.

61. Plottel, CS., Blaser, MJ. Microbiome and malignancy. Cell Host Microbe. 2011;10(4):324–35.

62. Heianza, Y., et al. Gut microbiota and risk of type 2 diabetes: The Japan Public Health Center-based Prospective Study. Scientific Reports. 2019;9(1):1 – 10.

63. Vrieze, A., Van Nood E., et al. Transfer of intestinal microbiota from lean donors increases insulin sensitivity in individuals with metabolic syndrome. Gastroenterology. 2012;143(4):913–6.e7.

64. Round, JL., Mazmanian, SK. The gut microbiota shapes intestinal immune responses during health and disease. Nat Rev Immunol. 2009;9(5):313–23.

65. Gensollen, T., Iyer, SS., et al. How colonization by microbiota in early life influences the development of the immune system. Science. 2016;352(6285):539–44.

66. Belkaid, Y., Hand, TW. The Role of the Microbiota in Immunity and Inflammation. Cell. 2014;157(1):121–41.

67. Round, JL., Lee, SM., et al. The Toll-like receptor two pathway establishes colonization by a commensal of the human microbiota. Science. 2011;332(6032):974–7.

68. Furusawa, Y., Obata, Y., et al. Commensal microbe-derived butyrate induces the differentiation of colonic regulatory T cells. Nature. 2013;504(7480):446–50.

69. Smith, PM., Howitt, MR., et al. The microbial metabolites, short-chain fatty acids, regulate colonic Treg cell homeostasis. Science. 2013;341(6145):569–73.

70. Atarashi, K., Tanoue, T., et al. Treg induction by a rationally selected mixture of Clostridia strains from the human microbiota. Nature. 2013;500(7461):232–6.

71. Kawai, T., Akira, S. The role of pattern-recognition receptors in innate immunity: update on Toll-like receptors. Nat Immunol. 2010;11(5):373–84.

72. Sanos, SL., Bui, VL, et al. RORgammat and commensal microflora are required for the differentiation of mucosal interleukin 22-producing NKp46+ cells. Nat Immunol. 2009;10(1):83–91.

73. Macpherson, AJ., McCoy, KD., et al. The immune geography of IgA induction and function. Mucosal Immunol. 2008;1(1):11–22.

74. Ivanov, II, Atarashi, K., et al. Induction of intestinal Th17 cells by segmented filamentous bacteria. Cell. 2009;139(3):485–98.

75. Frank, DN., St Amand AL., et al. Molecular-phylogenetic characterization of microbial community imbalances in human inflammatory bowel diseases. Proc Natl Acad Sci U S A. 2007;104(34):13780–5.

76. Fujimura, KE., Sitarik, AR., et al. Neonatal gut microbiota associates with childhood multisensitized atopy and T cell differentiation. Nat Med. 2016;22(10):1187–91.

77. Vatanen, T., Kostic, AD., et al. Variation in Microbiome LPS Immunogenicity Contributes to Autoimmunity in Humans. Cell. 2016;165(4):842–53.

78. Pamer, EG. Resurrecting the intestinal microbiota to combat antibiotic-resistant pathogens. Science. 2016;352(6285):535–8.

79. Desai, MS., Seekatz, AM., et al. A Dietary Fiber-Deprived Gut Microbiota Degrades the Colonic Mucus Barrier and Enhances Pathogen Susceptibility. Cell. 2016;167(5):1339–53.e21.

80. Ghosh, TS., et al. A Mediterranean diet intervention alters the gut microbiome in older people, reducing frailty and improving health status: the NU-AGE 1-year dietary intervention across five European countries. Gut. 2020;69(7):1218–28.

81. Singh, RK., Chang, HW., et al. The Influence of Diet on the Gut Microbiome and Its Implications for Human Health. J Transl Med. 2017;15(1):73.

82. David, LA., Maurice CF., et al. Diet rapidly and reproducibly alters the human gut microbiome. Nature. 2014;505(7484):559–63.

83. Zhang, Y., et al. A ketogenic diet induces time-dependent changes in microbiota and increases colonic permeability in healthy young mice. Acta Pharmaceutica Sinica B. 2020;10:497 – 510.

84. Windey, K., De Preter, V., et al. Relevance of protein fermentation to gut health. Mol Nutr Food Res. 2012;56(1):184–96.

85. Benedict, C., Vogel, H., et al. Gut microbiota and glucometabolic alterations in response to recurrent partial sleep deprivation in normal-weight young individuals. Mol Metab. 2016;5(12):1175–86.

86. Clarke, SF., Murphy, EF., et al. Exercise and associated dietary extremes impact on gut microbial diversity. Gut. 2014;63(12):1913–20.

87. Jin, Y., Wu, S., et al. Effects of Environmental Pollutants on Gut Microbiota. Environ Pollut. 2017;222:1–9.

88. Rook, GA. The hygiene hypothesis and autoimmune diseases. Clin Rev Allergy Immunol. 2012;42(1):5–15.

89. Gupta, VK., Kim, M., et al. A predictive index for health status using species-level gut microbiome profiling. Nat Commun. 2020;11(1):4635.

90. Chang, D., Gupta, VK., et al. The Gut Microbiome Wellness Index 2 enhances health status prediction based on gut microbiome taxonomic profiles. Nature Communications. 2024;15(1):7447.

91. Lozupone, CA., Stombaugh, JI., et al. Diversity, stability, and resilience of the human gut microbiota. Nature. 2012;489(7415):220–30.

92. Clarke, G, Stilling, RM., et al. Minireview: Gut microbiota: the neglected endocrine organ. Mol Endocrinol. 2014;28(8):1221–38.

93. Guinane, CM., Cotter, PD. Role of the gut microbiota in health and chronic gastrointestinal disease: understanding a hidden metabolic organ. Therap Adv Gastroenterol. 2013;6(4):295–308.

94. Slyepchenko, A., Maes, M., et al. Gut Microbiota, Bacterial Translocation, and Interactions with Diet: Pathophysiological Links between Major Depressive Disorder and Non-Communicable Medical Comorbidities. Psychother Psychosom. 2017;86(1):31–46.

95. Soliman, N., Kruithoff, C., et al. Small Intestinal Bacterial and Fungal Overgrowth: Health Implications and Management Perspectives. Nutrients. 2025;17(8).

96. Jacobs, C, Coss, AE., et al. Dysmotility and the use of proton pump inhibitors are independent risk factors for small intestinal bacterial and/or fungal overgrowth. Aliment Pharmacol Ther. 2013;37(11):1103–11.

97. Bowe, WP., Logan AC. Acne vulgaris, probiotics and the gut-brain-skin axis - back to the future? Gut Pathog. 2011;3(1):1.

98. de Magistris. L., Familiari V., et al. Alterations of the intestinal barrier in patients with autism spectrum disorders and in their first-degree relatives. J Pediatr Gastroenterol Nutr. 2010;51(4):418–24.

99. Spector, T. Food for Life: Your Guide to the New Science of Eating Well. UK: Vintage Publishing; 2024. 528 p.

100. Asnicar, F., Leeming, ER., et al. Blue poo: impact of gut transit time on the gut microbiome using a novel marker. Gut. 2021;70(9):1665–74.

101. Rezaie, A., Buresi, M., et al. Hydrogen and Methane-Based Breath Testing in Gastrointestinal Disorders: The North American Consensus. Am J Gastroenterol. 2017;112(5):775–84.

102. Bischoff, SC., Barbara, G., et al. Intestinal permeability--a new target for disease prevention and therapy. BMC Gastroenterol. 2014;14:189.

103. El-Salhy, M., Ystad, S. O., et al. The relation between gut microbiota and chronic constipation. World Journal of Gastroenterology. 2020;26(36):5757.

104. McDonald, D., Hyde, E., et al. American Gut: an Open Platform for Citizen Science Microbiome Research. mSystems. 2018;3(3).

105. De Filippis, F., Pellegrini, N., et al. High-level adherence to a Mediterranean diet has a beneficial impact on the gut microbiota and its associated metabolome. Gut. 2016;65(11):1812–21.

106. EFSA Panel on Dietetic Products N, and Allergies (NDA). Scientific Opinion on Dietary Reference Values for carbohydrates and dietary fibre. European Food Safety Authority (EFSA). 2010;8(3):75.

107. National Institute of Health (NIH). Dietary Reference Intakes: Energy, Carbohydrate, Fiber, Fat, Fatty Acids, Cholesterol, Protein, and Amino Acids. Washington DC., USA: National Academic Press; 2005.

108. Holscher, HD. Dietary fiber and prebiotics and the gastrointestinal microbiota. Gut Microbes. 2017;8(2):172–84.

109. Dalile, B., Van Oudenhove, L., et al. The role of short-chain fatty acids in microbiota-gut-brain communication. Nat Rev Gastroenterol Hepatol. 2019;16(8):461–78.

110. Macfarlane, S., Macfarlane, GT. Regulation of short-chain fatty acid production. Proc Nutr Soc. 2003;62(1):67–72.

111. Gibson, GR., Hutkins, R., et al. Expert consensus document: The International Scientific Association for Probiotics and Prebiotics (ISAPP) consensus statement on the definition and scope of prebiotics. Nat Rev Gastroenterol Hepatol. 2017;14(8):491–502.

112. Roberfroid, M. Prebiotics: The Concept Revisited. J Nutr. 2007;137 (Suppl 2):830s–7s.

113. Theuwissen, E., Mensink, RP. Water-soluble dietary fibers and cardiovascular disease. Physiol Behav. 2008;94(2):285–92.

114. Martínez-Villaluenga, C., Frías, J., et al. Functional relevance of prebiotic oligosaccharides in legumes. Foods. 2020;9(3).

115. Singh, B., Wani, AA., et al. The use of psyllium husk (Plantago ovata) for health and food applications. Food Reviews International. 2011;27(4):347 – 60.

116. Healey, G., Murphy, R., et al. Habitual dietary fiber intake influences gut microbiota response to an inulin-type fructan prebiotic: a randomized, double-blind, placebo-controlled, crossover, human intervention study. Br J Nutr. 2018;119(2):176–89.

117. Makki, K., Deehan, EC., et al. The Impact of Dietary Fiber on Gut Microbiota in Host Health and Disease. Cell Host Microbe. 2018;23(6):705–15.

118. Vojdani, A., et al. Lectins, agglutinins, and their role in autoimmune reactivities. Nutrients. 2019;11(6).

119. Cordain, L., Toohey, L., et al. Modulation of immune function by dietary lectins in rheumatoid arthritis. Br J Nutr. 2000;83(3):207–17.

120. Davis, CD., Milner, JA. Gastrointestinal microflora, food components, and colon cancer prevention. J Nutr Biochem. 2009;20(10):743–52.

121. Leite, AM., et al. Microbiological, technological, and therapeutic properties of Kefir: a natural probiotic beverage. Brazilian Journal of Microbiology. 2013;44(2):341 – 9.

122. Selma, MV., Espín, JC., et al. Interaction between Phenolics and Gut Microbiota: A Role in Human Health. J Agric Food Chem. 2009;57(15):6485–501.

123. Cardona, F., Andrés-Lacueva, C., et al. Benefits of Polyphenols on Gut Microbiota and Their Implications for Human Health. J Nutr Biochem. 2013;24(8):1415–22.

124. Spector, T. Food For Life: Your Guide to the New Science of Eating Well. Vintage, Penguin Random House Group UK; 2024. 528 p.

125. Aura, AM. Microbial metabolism of dietary phenolic compounds in the colon. Phytochem Rev. 2008;7:407 – 29.

126. Tzounis, X., Vulevic, J., et al. Flavanol monomer-induced changes to the human fecal microflora. Br J Nutr. 2008;99(4):782–92.

127. Parkar, SG., et al. Fruits and vegetables as a source of polyphenols and their effects on gut health. Curr Opin Clin Nutr Metab Care. 2013;16(6):679 – 85.

128. Dao, MC., Everard, A., et al. Akkermansia muciniphila and improved metabolic health during a dietary intervention in obesity: relationship with gut microbiome richness and ecology. Gut. 2016;65(3):426–36.

129. Qiao, Y., et al. Resveratrol ameliorates high-fat diet-induced insulin resistance and microbiota dysbiosis in mice. J Nutr Biochem. 2014;25(7):713 – 9.

130. Manach, C., Scalbert, A., et al. Polyphenols: food sources and bioavailability. Am J Clin Nutr. 2004;79(5):727–47.

131. Vauzour, D., Rodriguez-Mateos, A., et al. Polyphenols and human health: prevention of disease and mechanisms of action. Nutrients. 2010;2(11):1106–31.

132. González-Sarrías, A. Impact of flavonoids on gut microbiota composition and activity: a systematic review. J Agric Food Chem. 2017;65(24):4965 – 70.

133. Thursby, E., Juge, N. Introduction to the human gut microbiota. Biochem J. 2017;474(11):1823–36.

134. Sanders, ME., Merenstein, DJ. Probiotics and prebiotics in intestinal health and disease: from biology to the clinic. Nat Rev Gastroenterol Hepatol. 2019;16(10):605–16.

135. Hill C, Guarner F., et al. Expert consensus document. The International Scientific Association for Probiotics and Prebiotics consensus statement on the scope and appropriate use of the term probiotic. Nat Rev Gastroenterol Hepatol. 2014;11(8):506–14.

136. Marco, ML., Heeney, D., et al. Health benefits of fermented foods: microbiota and beyond. Curr Opin Biotechnol. 2017;44:94–102.

137. Wastyk, HC., Fragiadakis, GK., et al. Gut-microbiota-targeted diets modulate human immune status. Cell. 2021;184(16):4137–53.e14.

138. Tompkins, TA., Mainville, I., et al. The impact of meals on a probiotic during transit through a model of the human upper gastrointestinal tract. Benef Microbes. 2011;2(4):295–303.

139. Matuskova, Z., Anzenbacherova, E., et al. Administration of a probiotic can change drug pharmacokinetics: effect of E. coli Nissle 1917 on amiodarone absorption in rats. PLoS One. 2014;9(2):e87150.

140. Suez, J., Zmora, N., et al. Post-Antibiotic Gut Muc. Microbio. Reconstitution is impaired by probiotics and improved by αFMT. Cell. 2018;174(6):1406–23.e16.

141. Aguilar-Toala, JE. Postbiotics: An evolving term within the functional foods field. Trends in Food Science and Technology. 2018;75:105 – 14.

142. Klopper, KB., Deane, SM., et al. Aciduric Strains of Lactobacillus reuteri and Lactobacillus rhamnosus, Isolated from Human Feces, Have Strong Adhesion and Aggregation Properties. Probiotics Antimicrob Proteins. 2018;10(1):89–97.

143. Mu, Q., Tavella, VJ. Role of Lactobacillus reuteri in Human Health and Diseases. Front Microbiol. 2018;9:757.

144. Kim, MH., Kim, H. The Roles of Glutamine in the Intestine and Its Implications in Intestinal Diseases. Int. J. Mol. Sci. 2017; 18(5).

145. Monda, V., Villano, I., et al. Exercise Modifies the Gut Microbiota with Positive Health Effects. Oxid Med Cell Longev. 2017;2017:3831972.

146. Sohail, MU., Yassine, HM., et al. Impact of Phys. Exercise on Gut Microbio., Inflam., and the Patho. Of Metabolic Disorders. Rev Diabet Stud. 2019;15:35–48.

147. Jiang, Y., Guo, L., et al. Lactobacillus reuteri E9 Regulates Sleep Disorders Through Its Metabolite GABA. Front Biosci (Landmark Ed). 2025;30(6):39587.

148. Liu, B., Fan, L., et al. Gut microbiota regulates host melatonin production through epithelial cell MyD88. Gut Microbes. 2024;16(1):2313769.

149. Lee, HJ., Hong, JK., et al. Effects of Probiotic NVP-1704 on Mental Health and Sleep in Healthy Adults: An 8-Week Randomized, Double-Blind, Placebo-Controlled Trial. Nutrients. 2021;13(8).

150. Matsuda, Y., Ozawa, N., et al. Ergothioneine, a metabolite of the gut bacterium Lactobacillus reuteri, protects against stress-induced sleep disturbances. Transl Psychiatry. 2020;10(1):170.

151. Davis, W. Super Gut: A Four-Week Plan To Reprogram Your Microbiome, Restore Health, and Lose Weight. New York, USA: Balance publ.; 2023. 368 p.

152. Lin, Z., Jiang T., et al. Gut Microbiota and Sleep: Interaction Mechanisms and Therapeutic Prospects. Open Life Sci. 2024;19(1):20220910.

153. Williams, A., Diffenderfer, A., et al. Hands-on Cooking in Med. Schools: Diff. of a Prevention Education Innovation. Med. Science Educator. 2020;30(4):1591–8.

154. Eisenberg, DM., Myrdal Miller, A., et al. Enhancing Medical Education to Address Obesity: "See One. Taste One. Cook One. Teach One." JAMA Internal Medicine. 2013;173(6):470–2.

155. La Puma, J. What Is Culinary Medicine and What Does It Do? Population Health Management. 2016;19(1):1–3.

156. Staudacher, HM., Whelan, K. The low FODMAP diet: recent advances in understanding its mechanisms and efficacy in IBS. Gut. 2017;66(8):1517–27.

157. Magallanes, E., Sen, A., et al. Nutrition from the kitchen: culinary medicine impacts students' counseling confidence. BMC Med Educ. 2021;21(1):88.

158. Johnston, EA., Torres, M., et al. Integrating nutrition and culinary medicine into preclinical medical training. BMC Med Educ. 2024;24(1):959.

159. D'Adamo, CR., Workman, K., et al. Culinary Med. Training in Core Medical School Curriculum: Improved Med. Student Nutrition Knowledge and Confidence in Providing Nutrition Counseling. Am J Lifestyle Med. 2022;16(6):740–52.

160. Simmons, KB., et al. Combined hormonal contraceptives and antibiotics: A systematic review. Contraception. 2018;97(6):483 – 90.

161. Sobel, JD. Vulvovaginal candidosis. Lancet. 2007;369(9577):1961–71.

162. Centers for Disease Control and Prevention (CDC). Antibiotic Use in the United States, 2020 update: Progress & Opportunities. 2020.

163. Dethlefsen, L., Huse, S., et al. The pervasive effects of an antibiotic on the human gut microbiota, as revealed by deep 16S rRNA sequencing. PLoS Biol. 2008;6(11):e280.

164. Penumutchu, S., Korry, BJ., et al. Fiber supplementation protects from antibiotic-induced gut microbiome dysbiosis by modulating gut redox potential. Nat Commun. 2023;14(1):5161.

165. Theriot, CM., Koenigsknecht, MJ., et al. Antibiotic-induced shifts in the mouse gut microbiome and metabolome increase susceptibility to Clostridium difficile infection. Nat Commun. 2014;5:3114.

166. Leffler, DA., & Lamont, JT. Clostridium difficile infection. The New England Journal of Medicine. 2015;372(16):1539 – 48.

167. van Schaik, W. The human gut resistome. Philos Trans R Soc Lond B Biol Sci. 2015;370(1670):20140087.

168. Palleja, A., Mikkelsen, KH., et al. Recovery of gut microbiota of healthy adults following antibiotic exposure. Nat Microbiol. 2018;3(11):1255–65.

169. Jakobsson, HE., Jernberg, C., et al. Short-term antibiotic treatment has differing long-term impacts on the human throat and gut microbiome. PLoS One. 2010;5(3):e9836.

170. Jernberg, C., Löfmark, S., et al. Long-term ecological impacts of antibiotic administration on the human intestinal microbiota. Isme, J. (2007). 1(1), 56–66.

171. Kennedy, MS., Freiburger, A., et al. Diet outperforms microbial transplant to drive microbiome recovery in mice. Nature. 2025.

172. Sonnenburg, ED., Sonnenburg, JL. Starving our microbial self: the deleterious consequences of a diet deficient in microbiota-accessible carbohydrates. Cell Metab. 2014;20(5):779–86.

173. Allen, JM., Mailing, LJ., et al. Exercise Alters Gut Microbiota Composition and Funct. in Lean and Obese Humans. Med Sci Sports Exerc. 2018;50(4):747–57.

174. Shoaf, K., Mulvey, GL, et al. Prebiotic galactooligosaccharides reduce adherence of enteropathogenic Escherichia coli to tissue culture cells. Infect Immun. 2006;74(12):6920–8.

175. Li, P., Li, M., et al. Green Banana Flour Contributes to Gut Microbiota Recovery and Improves Colonic Barrier Integrity in Mice Following Antibiotic Perturbation. Front Nutr. 2022;9:832848.

176. Yang, S., Qiao, J., et al. Prevention and treatment of antibiotic-associated adverse effects through the use of probiotics: A review. J Adv Res. 2025;71:209–26.

177. Hempel, S., Newberry, SJ., et al. Probiotics for the prevention and treatment of antibiotic-associated diarrhea: a systematic review and meta-analysis. Jama. 2012;307(18):1959–69.

178. Ouwehand, AC., Salminen, S. Probiotics: an overview of beneficial effects. Antonie Van Leeuwenhoek. 2002;82(1-4):279–89.

179. Boyanova, L., Mitov, I. Co-administration of probiotics with antibiotics: why, when, and for how long? Expert Rev Anti Infect Ther. 2012;10(4):407–9.

180. Monteiro, CA., Cannon, G., et al. Ultra-processed foods: what they are and how to identify them. Public Health Nutr. 2019;22(5):936–41.

181. Bailey, DG., Dresser, G., et al. Grapefruit-medication interactions: forbidden fruit or avoidable consequences? CMAJ. 2013;185(4):309–16.

182. Cammarota, G., Ianiro, G., et al. International Consensus Conference on Stool Banking for Fecal Microbiota Transplantation in Clinical Practice. Gut. 2019;68(12):2111–21.

183. Kang, DW., Adams, JB., et al. Long-term benefit of Microbiota Transfer Therapy on autism symptoms and gut microbiota. Sci Rep. 2019;9(1):5821.

184. FDA. Important Safety Alert Regarding Use of Fecal Microbiota for Transplantation and Risk of Serious Adverse Reactions. U.S. Food & Drug Administration; 2022.

185. O'Toole, PW., Marchesi, JR., et al. Next-generation probiotics: the spectrum from probiotics to live biotherapeutics. Nat Microbiol. 2017;2:17057.

186. Jan, A., Bayle, P., et al. A consortium of seven commensal bacteria promotes gut microbiota recovery and strengthens the ecological barrier against vancomycin-resistant enterococci. Microbiome. 2025;13(1):129.

187. Zeevi, D., Korem, T., et al. Personalized Nutrition by Prediction of Glycemic Responses. Cell. 2015;163(5):1079–94.

188. Willyard, C. Microbiome therapy gains market traction. Nature Biotechnology. 2018;36(7):571 – 3.

189. Gopalakrishnan, V., Spencer, CN., et al. The gut microbiome modulates the response to anti-PD-1 immunotherapy in melanoma patients. Science. 2018;359(6371):97–103.

About the Author

The author is currently a Senior Lecturer in Physiology at RCSI-MUB. His career has included collaboration with numerous Functional Medicine practitioners, through which he gained direct insight into the vital roles that diet and environmental medicine play in patients' health and well-being. Recognizing the limited emphasis on nutrition in global medical curricula, the author was motivated to write a scientifically grounded, accessible book on the crucial relationship between the microbiome and health, and on how to care for our beneficial symbiotic microbiota partners, especially during antibiotic use.